# WHEN THE HUMOR IS
# GONE

## JAMES BEAN

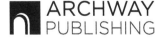
ARCHWAY PUBLISHING

Copyright © 2016 James H. Bean
Cover concept by James Kelly
Author photo © Robert Kley

All rights reserved. No part of this book may be used or reproduced by any means, graphic, electronic, or mechanical, including photocopying, recording, taping or by any information storage retrieval system without the written permission of the publisher except in the case of brief quotations embodied in critical articles and reviews.

Archway Publishing books may be ordered through booksellers or by contacting:

Archway Publishing
1663 Liberty Drive
Bloomington, IN 47403
www.archwaypublishing.com
1-(888)-242-5904

Because of the dynamic nature of the Internet, any web addresses or links contained in this book may have changed since publication and may no longer be valid. The views expressed in this work are solely those of the author and do not necessarily reflect the views of the publisher, and the publisher hereby disclaims any responsibility for them.

Any people depicted in stock imagery provided by Thinkstock are models, and such images are being used for illustrative purposes only.

Certain stock imagery © Thinkstock.

ISBN: 978-1-4808-0158-5 (sc)
ISBN: 978-1-4808-0160-8 (hc)
ISBN: 978-1-4808-0159-2 (e)

Library of Congress Control Number: 2013913055

Print information available on the last page.

Archway Publishing rev. date: 9/6/2016

*To the memory of
Muhammad Ali, Prince, and Malcolm X*

The greatness of a man is not in how much wealth he acquires, but in his integrity and his ability to affect those around him positively.

—Bob Marley

# TABLE OF CONTENTS

Preface . . . . . . . . . . . . . . . . . . . . . . . . . . . xi

Acknowledgments . . . . . . . . . . . . . . . . . . xvii

Introduction . . . . . . . . . . . . . . . . . . . . . xix

Chapter 1:  A Turning Point . . . . . . . . . . . . . 1

Chapter 2:  Finding Your Worth . . . . . . . . . . .15

Chapter 3:  Joys of Life . . . . . . . . . . . . . . . 41

Chapter 4:  The Crisis . . . . . . . . . . . . . . . 59

Chapter 5:  Who Depends on You? . . . . . . . . 67

Chapter 6:  If You Were Not Here . . . . . . . . . 79

| Chapter 7: | Leaving a Void | 87 |
| Chapter 8: | The Purpose of Life | 93 |
| Chapter 9: | Longevity | 107 |
| Chapter 10: | The Ones I Knew | 113 |
| Chapter 11: | Reasons for Doing It | 141 |
| Chapter 12: | Seeking Treatment | 153 |
| Chapter 13: | Discovering You | 161 |

# PREFACE

Suicide has intrigued me since I was a little boy. At that time I didn't understand what life events could bring a person to contemplate taking his or her own life. Most of my religious indoctrination focused on how life is precious and that I should honor God with my life. All I understood about death was its finality—that when we die, we cease to exist.

I recall attending a young boy's funeral when I was about six-years-old. It was at a time when the body was placed in the family's front parlor, and the wake was held in the family's home. I did not know this boy well. He lived near my cousin across town, and I used to play with him sometimes.

At his funeral, he lay motionless, his eyes closed, dressed in a black suit like grown men wore. I looked in curiosity and disbelief at his body in the casket. I could not believe that I would never see this boy alive again. My memories of him playing baseball or tag were replaced by the vision of his body lying in that casket.

Fast-forward about twenty-five years, and there was another young boy lying in a casket. This one was my little brother from the Big Brothers/Big Sisters agency. The agency had paired Timothy and me about four years earlier during my sophomore year in college. We enjoyed a great friendship, me acting as his mentor because his father left Timothy's family when he was seven-years-old.

I was living in Memphis when I received a telephone call at my office from the Big Brothers/Big Sisters case worker telling me Timothy had been involved in a shooting. She did not tell me at the time it was a suicide. I immediately grabbed my car keys and asked what hospital he was taken to so I could go and be with his family. There was a long pause, and the case worker said he didn't survive the shooting. I collapsed into my chair and began crying uncontrollably. I was shocked. Years later there would be a few other acquaintances of mine who committed suicide.

In the spring of 2004, I was confronted with my own depression and suicidal thoughts following my divorce and the death of my father a few months earlier. I shared excerpts of this book with a few friends, and they said I captured that critical moment of despair and hopelessness in describing my state of mind when I was on the precipice of taking my life. You will read my account of that day in chapter 1.

My underlying thought was that I didn't want to be on earth even one minute longer. I felt as if my head was centered in a metal vice and someone was turning it slowly, increasing the pain and pressure with each turn.

I was exhausted mentally and physically. There were days when I did not want to get out of bed; instead I would stay home, holed up, and not have to come into contact with anyone. I felt like a walking corpse, devoid of emotion, feeling, and desire. I just wanted to make the pain disappear.

For many years, I was promiscuous and used sex to fill the perceived void in my life. During the dark time in my life, however, I did not even entertain the thought of sex, although it was readily available to me. I lived in Las Vegas and was surrounded by women at both of my jobs. I did not even masturbate during this time because my depression was so great.

So there I was, failed marriage, struggling father, floundering career in comedy, and absolutely no one to talk to. I began visualizing the world without me. The truth was the world was going on with or without me. The truth was that someone, maybe more than one person, would mourn my passing and shed a few tears. The truth was those tears would dry, everyone would go back to living their lives, and my memory would soon fade.

I lost my brother and sister in a span of two years, and there was a time when I would think of them daily. Then it became less frequent, and later I would have passing thoughts even more infrequently. I wondered if that would happen with me.

I thought about the hierarchy of death and imagined that suicide was at the bottom, just under capital murder. Really, what could be lower than taking your own life? I wracked my brain and concluded that nothing could be.

I would become a statistic, particularly in Las Vegas where the suicide rate is uncommonly high. I thought of what the next day would be like, not for me, but for those who survived my death. I'd be the subject of water-cooler talk at work. There would be the irony of me being a comedian, bringing joy and laughter to so many when my own life was in turmoil and despair.

Overcome by a flood of emotion, the only thing that kept me from slicing my wrists that day was my love for my daughter.

Some people who have had a near-death experience say their entire life flashed before their eyes. I had a similar experience when I thought about committing suicide, but it wasn't my entire life that flashed before me; it was only the good parts that came to the forefront of my mind. It was as if my life was edited for this reason, and I saw a plethora of images flash before me like a Michael Bay movie, juxtaposed against the tremendous mental pain I was experiencing.

Amazingly, in that moment, just minutes before taking my life, I came to the realization that my life had been an incredible journey. I read a quote once about our lives being works of art, and we all start as a blank canvas. Through our own actions, we build a tapestry of memories, all compiled to make up a life.

I did not feel that my life was a master work of art like a Pablo Picasso painting, neither was it a tepid piece of art drawn by a four-year-old and placed on the refrigerator. The fact was, I had beaten the odds and was continuing to beat the odds with my life.

My life started in one of the worst ghettos in Providence, Rhode Island. I survived an abusive, absentee father. I was the product of a below average public school system, yet would earn a scholarship to law school. I had a failed marriage, but even it produced an exceptionally bright, beautiful daughter. I somehow blossomed from a quiet, shy little boy to an engaging, cerebral stand-up comedian.

I thought to myself, who the hell am I to decide to terminate this life? I had responsibilities, particularly to my daughter. I had always considered myself a generous person, but surely committing suicide would be the most selfish act of my entire life.

I was worthy of living. I said that to myself over and over. I did have joy in my heart, but I had to remind myself of those little things that made me happy. Those moments of pure joy that put a smile on my face were most important.

I thought about my goals as a stand-up comedian, the legacy I wanted to leave. I did not have grand visions of being on par with great comedians such as Richard Pryor, Rodney Dangerfield, Louis C.K. or George Carlin, but I still knew I could touch audiences and affect someone's life for just a few moments while I was on stage.

I thought about having purpose in my life. I knew I had lost my edge in the past few years, neglecting my wife, Christy, and my daughter, Soler. I had lost my way; I did not prioritize as I had in the past to reach my goals. I thought about the drive, purpose, and focus it took me to finish law school and pass the bar exam the first time. I was locked in at that time, committed to accomplishing this mammoth task.

I also realized in that moment that I needed to seek therapy immediately. I called my company's employee assistance program hotline shortly after this realization and was in therapy the next week. Seeking therapy was the most important decision I made at that time to turn my life around.

My ex-wife had always suspected that I suffered from depression because of my mood swings and unpredictable fits of anger. I could no longer deny that I had a problem, and I needed to seek professional help. I did, and I benefit from those sessions to this day. Ironically, it was later therapy sessions that led to the writing of this book.

I was starting to feel stagnant in my life. I hadn't accomplished much over the past few years, and I was fearful of depression seeping in again. My therapist asked me pointedly what I wanted to accomplish or what would make me feel that my life was moving forward. I told her that I wanted to write a book, so she told me to write a book.

Suicide, even with its stigma and dark undertones, was the only topic I wanted to address in my book. I was passionate about it because of what I had experienced earlier. My friend's husband committed suicide, and she and I talked extensively after that. I was one of the people she opened up to about her experience and dealing with the aftermath of her husband's death. We discussed his life, her guilt, and a multitude of issues surrounding his suicide. I wish we had taped our conversations because they were deep, thoughtful, and insightful. She is an amazing person who has done so much to overcome her husband's suicide and regain balance and perspective in her life.

My reason for writing this book is that I know there are others like me, like my friend's husband, who are suffering from severe depression and do not see a way out. They see suicide as a viable option to a temporary problem.

It is my hope that my words will encourage these people first to seek therapy from a licensed mental health professional. The stigma of seeking professional help for depression must be removed.  There are people in real pain, who are suffering daily from paralyzing depression.

Second, my book is intended to help suicide survivors. There are so many unanswered questions and feelings of guilt that suicide survivors have. I have dedicated one chapter of this book to those survivors and helping them cope with their loss.

I don't think there will be anything that I do in my life going forward that is more important than writing this book. That is not to say that I will not continue to grow and evolve.

This book is my love letter to the world, my legacy of care, hope, and empathy for those who are living under the gripping vice of depression.

# ACKNOWLEDGMENTS

I would like to thank Andrew Duggan for his financial contribution and steadfast support in helping me get this book published. I would also like to acknowledge my beautiful daughter, Soler Bean, for providing me the strength and inspiration for writing this book.

Special thanks to Steve Shakerian, Anthony Tricase, and my sister Sheila Baker for challenging me to write an honest, revealing, thought-provoking book on a difficult topic.

Finally, to my family and friends who inspire me in ways that I do not always acknowledge: you are my strength. Thank you.

# INTRODUCTION

Why was I lying in an empty tub with a razor blade to my wrists?

I was a golden boy of sorts, first in my family to earn an undergraduate degree. Graduated from law school and passed the bar exam on my first try. I was living the American dream: nice house, great career, beautiful five-year-old daughter.

Yet there I was on the brink of it all turning black like Tony Soprano on the final episode of *The Sopranos*. I was on the brink of being "that guy": seemingly happy-go-lucky, a kind word and smile for everyone he encountered.

Moreover, I was a comedian entertaining hundreds of people each night. Part of my craft was to make light of serious topics, twisting them and juxtaposing ideas so that people would laugh at the absurdity of it all.

What happens when the humor is gone? How could I possibly reconcile my job as a comedian making people laugh with the reality of dealing with severe depression that led to the suicidal state into which I was locked? I believe it was Shakespeare who coined the phrase "theatre of the absurd." There I was living it, sitting in the cold bathtub with my razor blades at the ready.

There was nothing heroic about what I was contemplating; rather, a cowardly act was about to happen. I was about to give a huge middle finger to the world, but did the world even care? In my manic, depressive state, did anything even matter? No. My death would be summed up in a three- or four-paragraph obituary. My family and friends would be dismayed that they didn't see the warning signs. In all honesty, I'd be nothing more than a sad statistic. It was fitting to become a statistic because at least I could fall into a category and be a part of something. I'd stopped feeling human months ago.

According to the Centers for Disease Control and Prevention (CDC), more than two million Americans contemplate suicide every year. More than one million attempt suicide each year and more than 40,000 succeed; more than one million succeed worldwide.

The American Foundation for Suicide Prevention (AFSP) estimates that there is a suicide in America every 13.7 minutes. Further, the AFSP says that 90 percent of suicides were diagnosed with a treatable psychiatric disorder.

A recent *USA Today* article pointed out that suicide deaths in the US military have tripled in recent years, averaging nearly thirty-three per month. And the CDC reports that the suicide rate among teenagers is the highest it has been in fifteen years.

It is these staggering statistics and my personal experience with a suicide attempt that prompted me to write this book.

While I am not a trained expert in the study of suicide or a licensed mental health professional, I am passionate about this subject. My personal experience with suicide stems from my own bout with suicidal thoughts several years ago and the number of friends who have had a close family member take his or her own life.

It was difficult for me to write this book because it is a delicate subject to discuss with anyone. I was continually challenged by my friends who wondered why I would want to write a book about such a dark subject. The only answer I could come up with was that I wanted to address a topic that I cared about. I wanted to share my thoughts about suicide with the notion that my words might encourage someone who may be contemplating suicide to reconsider that choice. My hope is that, by reading this book, people may have a better understanding of the suicidal mind and will explore the irrational thoughts and behavior behind it.

I have devoted several pages of this book to those friends and family members who have left a void in my heart—our hearts. I will explore the unanswered questions surrounding their decision to take their own lives and hopefully determine whether their suicides could have been avoided if people knew what to look for.

Based on the statistics cited earlier, my hope is that we all see the seriousness of this topic and how it is affecting so many families in this country and all over the world. I cannot think of a more numbing act than someone taking his or her own life. How does the suicidal mind work? Why do so many people succumb to their suicidal thoughts? How can we get more people to seek professional help when they are depressed or despondent?

These are some of the questions I raise and attempt to answer here. I recount my own battle with suicidal thoughts.

It was a bleak time for me, and I recall how depressed I was then. I will take you on my journey into my own emotional abyss, which culminated in a day that I will never forget.

Obviously, I have overcome my own suicidal thoughts because I am writing this book. Reliving that downward spiral has been painful yet in some ways rewarding. I believe completely in the indomitable human spirit. I feel we are like other animals; instinctually, we want to survive. Therefore, I am perplexed by the idea that anyone would want to commit suicide and at the number of people who accept suicide as a viable option.

I hope that as you read through this book, you feel my compassion, empathy, and sheer passion for this topic. Suicide is not easy to discuss because of the stigma that surrounds it. Not many people admit to having suicidal thoughts for fear of being judged and deemed mentally unstable.

In my research, which includes many discussions with family members and friends, over the course of their lives, most people have at least contemplated suicide. If we are to have serious discussions about this topic, we need to take suicide off the list of taboo subjects. More research and study is needed to reduce the number of suicides, particularly in the armed forces, where it is most prevalent among our valued service men and women.

This book is intended for anyone who has considered suicide. It is also intended for people who may know someone who is contemplating self-harm. And finally, it is my intent to help those who have had a close friend or family member commit suicide. Many times those friends and family members are left with unanswered questions and a void that can never be filled. The grief, pain, and guilt can be unbearable. Death is inevitable for all of us; we do not have to hasten it with our own hands.

## CHAPTER 1

# A TURNING POINT

*Remember, you're braver than you believe, stronger than you seem, and smarter than you think.*

—Christopher Robin

A series of events brought me to the place where I considered suicide, but the tipping point was my divorce. I knew I was heading for divorce even though my wife and I tried couples therapy, and I made desperate attempts to try to keep our marriage whole. It didn't register with me at the time, but my wife arranged for us to be separated nearly a year. She did this under the guise of guiding my daughter's budding acting career. We were living in Reno at the time, and had just purchased a house.

She and my daughter moved to L.A., where I set them up in an apartment in a nice neighborhood just west of TCL Theatre. Many of our friends and family commented about how pretty our daughter was, and they thought she had a chance to be successful acting with her bubbly personality. I was skeptical because I knew how competitive it was in L.A., and felt my daughter would be one of thousands of children trying to get work. My wife was the "stage mom" in our family.

I didn't enjoy the time away from my wife and daughter. I lived as if I was single, going out to clubs, meeting women and having affairs. When I did visit them in L.A., we would argue about the usual issues couple argue about; money, parenting, and sex. I was exhausted. I knew in my heart that my marriage was at the brink, but I wanted to hold on for appearances. I did not want to look bad in front of my family and friends. My stint in Reno, Nevada was over, and I was moving back to Las Vegas. I contracted to buy a house and my wife indicated she was willing to give our marriage more try.

Our living conditions at the time were unstable. I signed a year contract to work in a production show called X Burlesque. My producer allowed me to rent out his home until he found a buyer. His home was gorgeous, specious and had a pool. The only negative is that it was about 25 miles from the strip in Henderson, NV. There was no easy route to the strip, if I took the surface streets it was a 45 minute drive. If I took the highway, it was about 30 minutes but the expressway looped around the city. My producer's home sold after two months and we had to move to an extended stay hotel.

It was there that my wife made the final decision to divorce me. Now I was faced with moving into a home by myself that I purchased for my family. I could not get out of the contract, so I had to go through with the home purchase. I did not want to own a home without a family. I felt like everything was crashing down on me. Nothing seemed right to me, I was losing my family, and I felt more alone than I ever have in my life.

I began to keep a mental checklist of what I needed to do before I ended my life. I did not want to provide any warning signs regarding my plans, so I avoided giving away valuables or money to friends and family.

I continued to go to work at a major Las Vegas hotel where I performed stand-up comedy, but I was just going through the motions. I had never felt such numbness in my life. I felt detached from my work, friends, and family. Yet somehow I did a great job of hiding how I felt, even though all the signs of my depression were there.

Prior to this, I thought I was a happy person for the most part. I had worked hard at being a happy person. I did my best to create opportunities for myself to be happy. I prided myself on being the type of person who engaged well with others. But after my divorce, I began to question my life, eventually becoming detached from it.

I had always tried to do the right thing, to follow a certain path to success and happiness. In fact, by the age of eight, I had already mapped out what I was going to do with my life. After high school, I would enlist in the army. Once I left the army, I would attend the University of Memphis in Tennessee and try out for its basketball team.

I followed through on my goals, almost in a paint-by-numbers fashion. However, given all that I had accomplished, I eventually reached a crossroads in my life and seriously contemplated suicide.

Now that I had decided to commit suicide, I knew I had to write a note explaining my decision. Surprisingly, that was not as difficult as I thought it would be. I simply wanted to address the people who were most important to me: my daughter, mom, and sisters. As you will see in the actual suicide note (described later in this chapter), I did not include any friends because I wasn't especially close to anyone at the time.

I recall years earlier having read several suicide notes in a book about the subject called *The Suicidal Mind* by Edwin S. Shneidman. It was eerie to read actual suicide notes because of how personal each one was. They often detailed what each person was going through. I found that I liked reading about suicide and the psychological aspects of the act. It was hard for me to check out books on suicide from the library and even harder to buy one at the bookstore. It feels weird carrying around a book like that in your hand. You think people are looking at you at the checkout or fear someone will see you with it.

At this point, I did not care about much of anything, but I needed to understand what was happening to me. I wanted to know why I felt so depressed. I read several books about suicide, most about suicide prevention and others exploring the psychological aspects of the suicidal mind. Two notable books I read were *Veronika Decides to Die* by Paulo Coelho, and *Suicide* by Emile Durkheim, George Simpson and John Spaulding. According to everything I read, suicide was the last resort for most people suffering from depression or other psychological disorders or pressures.

My divorce hit me hard. I'd never really failed at anything, but here I was getting divorced after just six years of marriage. My wife and I had a five-year-old daughter, and I felt I had failed her as a father because my marriage fell apart. As a result, I began to immerse myself in my work. I became blurry eyed during my day job working in customer service support for a major casino and totally exhausted at night after doing my comedy gig.

In my mind, nothing was going right. I did not have the right job, the right house, the right amount of money, the right car, or the right girl. In fact, after the divorce, I had no girl at all.

Absolutely nothing felt right to me during this period of my life. I took on a zombie-like appearance: somber, always serious, and rarely laughing or smiling. This was a vast departure from my usual friendly demeanor. I was not the life of the party or the alpha dog in social situations, but you knew I was in the room. There was an absence of life, of passion, of purpose. It was the most frightening feeling I'd ever had in my life.

The thing I remember most about the moment I decided to commit suicide was that I did not want to be on this earth any longer. I did not want to be on this big blue marble, with all its problems and seemingly unending drama—not a minute or second longer.

I sat there in my home, disconnected from everyone. I was lost in my perceived failures and my despair. Other than my daughter, I did not feel connected to anyone, which is what made my decision to kill myself so easy. "Who would miss me?" I thought. Sure my mom and sisters loved me, but I had not lived at home for more than twenty-five years. I even felt disconnected from them. Except for a few obligatory phone calls on holidays and birthdays, we had little contact since I had left home. Killing myself that day just felt right, as normal as going to the movies or out to dinner.

I simply had no purpose. Sadly, my daughter's future and well-being was not enough to keep me from the thought of killing myself. Even when I considered not being there to raise my daughter, it was not enough to change my intent. I felt she would be fine. I assumed my ex-wife would remarry; therefore, my daughter would still have a father figure in her life. Furthermore, I honestly felt I could no longer add value to her life. I fully believed that I had nothing to offer my daughter or the world. I felt the world would be better off without me. It was time to leave it all behind.

Ironically, years earlier, I had often contemplated what a selfish act suicide was. I had often debated this with my friends. In the past, I did not have any compassion for those who had chosen this route.

Prior to my decision to take my own life, I knew four people who committed suicide: my boss's teenage son, a young man to whom I was a big brother, a coworker at the showroom where I performed, and another coworker from years earlier. Each haunted me in different ways. I attended all four memorial services, and I cried at them all. My emotions and reactions were different at each funeral. I was in sheer shock at my boss's son's funeral. My boss showed strength and dignity throughout the service, but I knew he was devastated. I could not fathom what he must have felt burying his child.

My emotions during Timothy's funeral were different. I was his big brother, a position I valued. I sat at his memorial with a sense of remorse and guilt. I felt I had failed him in some way. The three years spent as his mentor and big brother were fruitless to me because of this tragic end. I was angered at my friend Cisco's funeral because I knew he had a young son, and I couldn't believe anyone would leave their child like that no matter what the circumstances were. My colleague Dave, who took his own life also left a child. I just remember thinking I'd sit with him in staff meetings and I would never see him again.

The death of the young man to whom I was big brother was perhaps the most devastating to me. I was his mentor, and I wondered where I had gone wrong in our relationship.

At my boss's son's funeral, I was baffled as to why a teenager would want to take his own life. When I was his age, I felt invincible. Death did not even seem possible to me at that time.

I was told by others who worked with him that my coworker from the showroom had been suffering greatly from depression and that his wife treated him terribly. I had hung out with him a couple of times, and he seemed like a normal person with his share of normal problems.

My coworker from years earlier had a family. He apparently killed himself because he was involved in a love triangle. I did not know him that well; I only saw him in a few meetings at work. Again, he seemed by all appearances to be a happy, content person.

After these four suicides, I thought if I went through with my attempt, I would be one of "those people." I would be the guy whom people talked about at the water cooler. They would talk about how I seemed so normal and happy. My family would have been shocked because, in their minds, I had overcome and accomplished so much in my life. People who disliked me would be vindicated because, in the end, my suicide would indicate my flawed character and unstable condition.

I was incapable of being trusted with my own life. You would think if a person was about to leave this world, the last thing on his or her mind would be what others thought of him or her.

I flipped back and forth between emotions. I told myself that I did care what others thought of me, particularly my mother and daughter. My mother had been crushed years earlier. She had already lost two of her children: my sister to murder and my brother to AIDS. I would be the third child she would have to bury. But I had convinced myself that my death would be different.

Unlike my siblings, I chose not to be here any longer; therefore, it was okay. I loved my daughter, but I reasoned that that was not enough to make me stay. She was a wonderful little girl, so smart and fun to be around. Unfortunately, I had lost the desire to hear her joyful laughter. My mind was in a horrible place, a place I never imagined I would be.

My suicide note was written, so now I just needed to kill myself. I had plenty of pills in the house, but they were mostly aspirin and cold medicines. I was sure mixing over-the-counter pills with alcohol would do the trick. Then I deduced they would not be strong enough.

Next I decided I should slit my wrists. I read somewhere that for this to be effective, I needed to slash my wrists up and down along the vein and not across it. Nah that would be too messy. Now I started thinking about who would have to clean up the mess.

I contemplated doing both: taking pills to sedate myself and then slitting my wrists. But then the thought of who would clean up the mess entered my mind again. You would be surprised at the type of random thoughts that enter your mind in this mental state. Even though I would be dead soon, I made sure my house was clean and orderly. Now I began to question if I was comfortable messing up the house I had just cleaned.

I began to think of who would possibly discover my body. I did not want it to be my daughter or ex-wife. The thought of how a good friend had found his sister's body after she committed suicide flooded my brain. I recalled how deeply it had affected him. I questioned how I could do this to those I loved.

In the end, as I sat with my suicide note, pills, and razor blades within arm's length, I could not do it. I began to rethink my dilemma. The strain on my mother would be too much.

I realized my daughter was the most precious thing in my life. I wanted to see her grow up and have children. I began to remember the dire statistics of children whose parents committed suicide; many of those children followed suit and also committed suicide.

I began to change my mind. As these thoughts came in waves, I decided to live another day. With each passing day, I decided to live another week, and then another month, and finally another year. It was not easy. In many ways I felt like an alcoholic or a drug addict who needed to complete a twelve-step program. It was literally one day at a time.

Shortly thereafter, I began to see a therapist. I mentioned my suicidal tendencies only in passing, as if everyone has probably thought about it at one time or another. I continued to live from day to day, building on my desire to live as each day passed.

Life places many pressures and demands on us: work, children, relationships, financial burdens, illness, and uncertainty, to name just a few. How we cope with these pressures reveals our character. The one certainty we have is that life's challenges will be with us until we die—hopefully of natural causes.

There are many instances where we feel overwhelmed, and suicidal tendencies can rule our thoughts. To be fair, suicide is an option—fortunately most agree not the best one. But when the suicidal mind takes hold, it can appear to be the only option. Learning to squelch that thought is the hard part.

I have concluded that one of the best ways to avoid a suicidal thought is to create a purpose for your life. Find a way to stay connected to those who are important to you. I recently had a philosophical discussion with a friend. The question at hand was, what is the purpose of life? I answered to live our lives. I still believe this to be true. Just get up every morning and live the life that is placed in front of you. It will not always be an easy one. But when you have a bad day, you will usually find the problem you had is better by the next day. Just get through the bad one.

I think anyone can find purpose in life. For me, purpose is anything you do, religious or otherwise, that enriches your life or the lives of others. I believe if you find that calling or purpose, everything else falls into place and you can enjoy life's pleasures. There are many simple pleasures in life, and I think if you search long enough, you will find one or more purposes or pleasures that suit your needs. Life is worth sustaining.

Building meaningful relationships can help give each of us purpose. My most cherished relationship is with my daughter. It has not always been easy. At best, it is a work in progress. In fact, it has been a work in progress for sixteen years.

I am always amazed at how close we have become. I used to joke with my daughter, when she was a toddler, that she was the only person who understood me. To this day, I still believe she is the only person who truly understands me. In addition to my daughter, I have established great friendships over the years.

Since the thoughts of that terrible day, I have committed myself to building and sustaining those relationships. My current inner circle of friends is the best I have had in years. My friends challenge me, support me, and kick me in the butt when I need it. They are a perfect blend of tough love, compassion, and understanding. Together, my family and friends make me a better person. My family as I see it consists of my mother Matilda, my daughter Soler, my older sister Sheila, and my two younger sisters Marie and Pamela. I don't consider myself close to my sisters, mostly because of the physical distance between us. I have lived away from all of them for decades. I do call each of them on holidays or when there are major life events happening with me or my daughter.

My daughter spends summers in Rhode Island, and seems to enjoy being with my sisters. I want her to forge a strong bond with them so she doesn't rely solely on me for support and guidance. I want her to have a strong mind, and make sound decisions. Ironically, my daughter fought her own bout with depression in recent years. She wrote to her mother about crippling depression over a two-year period. We immediately placed her in counseling, and by all accounts her demeanor and attitude have improved. Her letter cut straight to my heart because it was so similar to the feelings I felt years earlier.

Despite how glorious the human brain is, our mind can deceive us. The mind determines how we perceive ourselves and the world. The mind never shuts off, so it continually floods us with thoughts, even in our sleep. Many times these thoughts are unfiltered, meaning we do not learn to understand where they come from. Were they from a negative influence or a positive one? These thoughts often come in waves and can seem never-ending.

Our thoughts can be inspirational, bringing us great joy and a sense of accomplishment. But some thoughts can be harmful, causing us to see ourselves in a seemingly unfavorable light. It is those thoughts that must be controlled or at least viewed through a different lens.

We may not always feel good about ourselves, but it is critical that we see ourselves realistically. Learn your weaknesses in order to control them. Find what makes you happy and allow that happiness to be a part of your life, despite what others may think. We must learn to acknowledge our humanity and our frailty, accept who we are, and be OK with it.

This is the letter I wrote when I was contemplating suicide:

To my mother, who was the best mother a kid could have, I am sorry. I should have been stronger, Ma. I am sorry to leave you with this burden after all you have been through. I do not expect you to understand, but please know that you did a great job raising all of us. I am just very tired of living. You provided me with love and support to be successful in this life, and I thank you for that. I am sorry for this pain and all the pain that you have had to endure over the years. I hope you can forgive me.

To my dearest Soler, who is my best friend and partner in life. You were the only reason for me to live, and I thank you for your pure heart. Soler, you will never understand why Daddy did this. I want you to pursue all of life's dreams and remember that I love you. You have many memories of me to reflect on. You will always be my little Nooble. You represent all that is right in the world. I love you.

Sheila, I am sorry that I let you down. You were the only one who sensed that I was depressed, and I could not bring myself to tell anyone else. I know you are disappointed. I always loved you for your strength and ability to fight through tough times. I was too tired to fight. I hope that you will look after Soler for me. I wished we would have talked more. I wished that we had shared more of our lives. Thank you for all that you have done for me.

Pamela, this pains me because I know that you have been proud of what I have been able to accomplish in this life. I am asking that you do one thing for me, and that is be there for your children. I know I have not always been there for you, and I am sorry. I hope you can forgive me.

Marie, my dearest Marie: I love you so much. You have always had the greatest demeanor and navigated life with a smile on your face. You are funnier than I could ever be, and you are a great mother. I am so proud of Marquis and Jeneara. You could always make me laugh, even during the toughest times. I know that my death will hit you the hardest, and I hope you will find it in your heart to forgive me; I have just been very tired and simply cannot do this anymore. Please stay in touch with Soler. She loves you so much. When she talked about seeing Jack, she really was talking about you. You always listened to her stories and she loves talking to you.

To my nieces and nephews, whom I love: I never did enough for any of you and for that I am sorry. I do not think that any of you realize how hard this life is and what you will need to sacrifice to succeed. Make your own path and never give up on your dreams. You can do whatever you want to in life, just live with a passion for it.

All of you have provided me with a certain joy and happiness. Do not look upon my death as a tragic ending. I have always made my own decisions in life and while this decision will not be popular, it is mine. I love you all.

James Bean
February 11, 2004

## CHAPTER 2

# FINDING YOUR WORTH

*The grand essentials of happiness are: something to do, something to love, and something to hope for.*

—*Allan K. Chalmers*

"Just who the hell do you think you are?"

That was the question posed to me by the CEO of the security protection firm where I worked in 1992. The question jolted me, and I did not answer it immediately, so he shouted the question at me again and demanded that I answer it.

I sat in stunned silence thinking there was no right answer, and I did not appreciate the spirit in which the question was being asked.

I had declined a promotion in the company, which would have made me the director of marketing. It was a job I felt ill equipped to handle, given my limited background and inexperience just coming out of college. I had worked for the company during college as the night dispatcher and had seen the revolving door of people getting fired seemingly within weeks of getting hired for the marketing position.

But the question was posed to me because I had just graduated law school and passed the Tennessee bar on the first try. I had accepted a position as the company's compliance officer and enjoyed that role. So I wasn't sure whether the CEO was trying to goad me into saying something that could be considered disrespectful or insubordinate.

My first thought was to tell him I was an attorney. Again, the question was asked in the spirit of who was I to turn down an opportunity that had been presented to me. Honestly, I felt I was a person who had just graduated law school, passed the bar, and had options. Because I had that piece of paper, my law degree, I could say no to a host of offers because my world was about to expand.

The question challenged my worth as a human being. I did not appreciate it at that time and, in retrospect, should have resigned right there on the spot. But I was paralyzed by the question. I was stunned it was even asked of me, but there I was with no reply at the ready.

I felt disrespected but had no recourse because it was the CEO of the company. He was smarter than me, right? He was correct in his thinking, right? He had every right to challenge my worth as a human being, right? I had no answer at the time to the question before me. If I had the courage at the time I would have told him I'm James Bean! That's who the fuck I am, I'm James Bean!

I felt my boss was questioning my value in asking me that question. It is my firm belief that every person placed on this earth has value. I further believe that from the time we are born, there is a constant assault on our self-esteem, particularly an attack on our worthiness to be here.

There are many factors that shape who we ultimately become, for instance, financial and emotional stability. Consider a newborn child. Every child deserves the best life possible. That newborn, in my opinion, is invaluable. As a father, I feel a child's worth is found in the potential to create that special life. Children come into this world with so much promise and hope, but it is up to their parents to give them proper guidance.

Furthermore, it is important to understand that our birth established our worth or value. I realize I may be creating controversy by stating we have worth from the day we are born, but I am not measuring our worth in the terms of monetary value. Our worth in that sense is invaluable. I am talking about our contribution to life. Bottom line: We all have worth.

As we get older, we realize the key for survival is establishing an identity and self-worth. This is where life can get complicated. I heard an interesting quote once comparing today's youth with children born decades ago. Children today want to be rich and famous, whereas children decades earlier wanted to be something meaningful, such as a doctor, dentist, or lawyer. I think this distinction is important to contemplate given the rise of pseudo-celebrities such as Paris Hilton and Kim Kardashian, who have not accomplished anything but whose notoriety are widespread. Kardashian's popularity has always escaped me because her big debut on the national stage was a sex tape with a D list talent.

Men and women of my generation—the baby boomers—dreamed of becoming firefighters, lawyers, doctors, dentists, or police officers, for instance. And why not since these are all noble pursuits? Today, the media, particularly television, have presented children with a false sense of accomplishment. We live in a celebrity-worshiping culture with little or no consideration for why a person is famous. In my opinion, being famous or well-known is not an accomplishment and only adds to the difficulty of finding yourself. For example, Charles Manson is famous and has been the subject of countless books, documentaries, and even a popular movie, *Helter Skelter*. But being like Manson is not something to strive for, or emulate.

So are you famous and accomplished just because you are on television? Many children today would say yes because millions of people can see you on television, therefore you must be important. My own self-worth has been defined by accomplishments, such as graduating high school, finishing a four-year stint in the army, graduating from college, and finally finishing law school and passing the Tennessee Bar exam. I look back on each of those accomplishments proudly. I felt I had to earn a place in society. I continue to earn my place in society by being a good father, comedian, employee, and citizen.

In my mind, my past accomplishments have added value to my life. While most of my accomplishments are rooted in academic achievement, other people add value to their lives by accomplishing goals in other areas, such as through military service, sports, volunteering in the community, or parenting. There are thousands of people like me who have never been on television or the cover of a major magazine or newspaper, yet they are accomplished.

Self-worth to me means having a series of accomplishments, big and small, which in turn make up a person's life as a whole. When there are no accomplishments, then a person cannot help but feel inadequate compared with their peers. In the absence of accomplishments, there may be feelings of despair or being less compared with others. This feeling of inadequacy can lead to depression and eventually being suicidal. Finding a passion for life, setting goals, and pursuing them relentlessly are key to realizing your full potential.

I do not think a person must be unrealistic or have delusions of grandeur, but you must be your own biggest fan and supporter. Who else will sing your praises greater than you? What I mean is there is no harm in feeling you are great. This is not to say that you should not have an accurate read on who you are. I think you have to be mindful about developing an overinflated ego.

I think it is critical to see yourself in a positive light. Be your own public relations agent. Think of it this way: we constantly promote ourselves, whether it is trying to win the hand of a beautiful woman (or man) or landing our dream job. We constantly need to sell ourselves. Any salesperson worth his or her salt will tell you that one of the biggest factors in selling anything is to believe in the product. You need to believe in yourself to sell yourself; it is that simple.

In selling yourself, it is important to understand and accept external feedback. It may or may not mirror how we perceive ourselves. An example that comes to mind is the contestants who are dismissed during the auditions for the popular talent show *American Idol*. It amazes me how many of these people really believe they have talent and the judges just do not see it or they are oblivious to their potential. Many of these contestants do have delusions of grandeur and will continue to fail in life because they reject any external criticism as invalid.

Rejection is never easy, whether it happens in front of millions of people or in front of just a few. It always feels awful. You can feel rejected from something as benign as asking a woman to dance at a nightclub and she says "No, thank you. I'll pass." There is always that long walk back to your table, shoulders slumped and ego bruised. It may seem as though everyone heard the conversation, and every eye in the club is watching you. You feel that you just want to disappear.

There are many traps to playing the self-esteem game, and many are internal. I remember a particular session with my therapist during a rough time in my life. Even though I had accomplished all the goals mentioned earlier, I still felt inadequate. I felt my career had stalled. I was not making the money I thought I should be making. In my mind, I thought I should have saved a few thousand dollars in the bank, apart from my 401K. The reality was, one day after I had just been paid, I had only $104 left in my checking account. My therapist reassured me that in the grand scheme of things I was doing just fine. My therapist provided me with a new perspective.

The therapist then took me through an exercise that dealt with the word "should." The exercise helped me understand how damaging the word should can be. Should oftentimes takes the place of "is not," for example, "This is not the way it is." When we look at the word should this way, we build up certain expectations and then fall short. We somehow process this as a failure. Again, this is a dangerous way to process where we are in life.

I can only imagine how the word should works inside the suicidal mind. If the catalyst for committing suicide is a failed relationship, the person may feel he or she should still be loved by an ex-boyfriend or ex-girlfriend, interpreted as meaning he or she is not loved by the ex. If the turning point is a financial failure, the person may feel he or she should have $100,000 in the bank, interpreted as there is not $100,000 in the bank.

You can see how viewing your life by what you think should happen vs. what is actually happening can put you in a depressive state. Using the word should can damage your self-esteem if you internalize should as a failure.

There is a wonderful passage from the Bible Philippians 4:12 that says, "I have learned to be content in all circumstances." I love this quote because it speaks to the writer's ability to be complete as a person, no matter what fate should befall him. Think of the power of this statement, which diminishes the "should" that may be present. The author retains his power no matter what external forces are present.

Sometimes external forces try to diminish us; this can be our parents, siblings, coaches, friends, clergy, or the talking heads on television. I believe that our parents have the greatest influence on our self-esteem for the mere fact we spend most of our childhood and young adulthood with them.

Some parents are nurturing and encouraging to the point where their children believe they can become anything they want to be. I am in favor of encouraging children this way but always within reason. However, some parents damage their children's confidence so badly that they feel they are worthless and not capable of accomplishing anything.

From childhood to young adulthood, most children receive external messages regarding their self-worth: "You are smart." "You are a great athlete." "You are clumsy." "You are dumb." Young minds likely internalize all these messages; they certainly have the propensity to become self-fulfilling prophecies. Parents have a duty to reinforce good behaviors by providing children with positive feedback. After all, according to Aristotle, "We are what we repeatedly do."

External messages, including media messages that kids receive, can be overwhelming. Negative messages were at the root of the Columbine High School shootings in 1999. The two students responsible for the shootings, Dylan Klebold and Eric Harris, were reportedly bullied unmercifully at their school. They were part of a fringe group that was labeled "goths" because they listened to heavy-metal music and wore black clothing. They could no longer take the stress and strain of going to school and were determined to make the psychological pain stop by any means necessary. The two social outcasts formulated a plan to get even with those students who were part of the "in crowd," namely jocks and popular kids. From all accounts, these two kids planned a double suicide, which expanded to killing several people in the end. It is important to have an awareness of the devaluation game, or bullying, which some people play skillfully.

I think this can occur in situations where we should feel most protected, for instance, in a committed relationship. It is amazing to me how a couple's feelings change on a dime when the issue of divorce or separation comes to the surface. A couple can coexist for many years, caring, nurturing, and showing love toward each other. Unfortunately, once they decide to terminate the relationship, one or both are demonized and suddenly neither has any intrinsic worth.

I experienced this phenomenon in my own marriage and was surprised when I realized how hateful some of my e-mails were to my ex-wife following our divorce. She and I deliberately lobbed verbal assaults at each other that were intended to cause psychological damage.

Teachers can sometimes plant seeds of doubt in our minds too. I recall reading *The Autobiography of Malcolm X*, where he recounted how a grade-school teacher once asked him what he wanted to be when he grew up. Malcolm X, without hesitation, told his teacher he wanted to be a lawyer. The teacher replied that being a lawyer was not a realistic goal for a Negro. The teacher instead suggested Malcolm think about becoming a carpenter.

I recall a similar instance when I entered seventh grade. I had previously attended a private school through sixth grade before I transferred to a public school. The guidance counselor at the public school, without even looking at my academic record from my previous school, suggested I start with a remedial-level reading class. I honestly felt he was making this snap assessment because I was black. It was never suggested that I take an aptitude or proficiency test to determine my reading level. Sometimes I laugh out loud when I think to myself that the counselor may have been right, considering I did not even know what the word "remedial" meant at the time. Nevertheless, I knew that I was reading at an eighth- or ninth-grade level.

This was not the only experience of racism I had in a school setting. All of my life, teachers, professors, and guidance counselors made assumptions based on my race, assuming I was not at the academic level of my peers.

There are many other areas where our self-esteem comes under assault. It would be dangerous to underestimate how religion may play a role in some suicides. However, statistics show that people who follow some religious idealism commit suicide less frequently than atheists.

Many religions are based on the common tenant that there is an all-powerful and all-knowing God. Furthermore, some religious dogma rests on the idea of predestination, meaning that God has already mapped out a grand plan that cannot be altered since it was written centuries before your birth. Other Christian sects do promote free will, which I tend to agree with in theory.

I have always found this theory troubling on many levels. If this is true, it likely causes people to take a more reactive approach to their lives. I am sure you have heard a few of these refrains from people who believe in God: "It is all in God's hands" or "God willing" or "God wants us to have this child" or perhaps "It is all in God's plan." Such refrains are quite chilling to me because it supposes that we have no control over our lives or our circumstances. The notion is that God determines our fate.

The danger in accepting this as true is, if we believe someone or something else controls our life, it absolves us of any personal responsibility. If you do not feel responsible for your life, then your life is worthless. And anyone who believes their life is worthless runs the risk of internalizing negative thoughts, which could result in suicidal thoughts or harmful actions.

Sin, another aspect of religion, also plays a part in suicide. Some religions teach us that we are born in sin, meaning we are somehow stained the second we emerge from the womb. How can a person be flawed at birth? Feelings of guilt and worthlessness directly descend from the idea of sin. It is not necessary to list what may be considered sin because the list would be prohibitive, expanding well beyond the Ten Commandments.

A person potentially may feel like a failure or have feelings of guilt if he or she has sinned. I used to harbor those feelings until I realized life is one long lesson. No matter how old we are, we can—and will—make mistakes or sin. The key is to learn from our mistakes. Nonetheless, given my age, education, and life experiences, it is hard for me to believe that I can still make mistakes.

The fact that sin can be forgiven does not quell the notion that a person has failed by sinning in the first place. It is this feeling of failure that can have a lasting effect on an individual, causing him or her to feel inadequate or, worse, not worthy of living.

Gaining a positive image of self-worth is critical for avoiding feelings of despair and depression. The most effective way to gain self-esteem and a sense of self-worth is through accomplishment. Even if your accomplishments aren't on par with Oprah Winfrey or Bill Gates, you still have a body of work about which you can be proud. Remember, much of your worth is wrapped in your achievements or even your potential. It is what you have the ability to create that is important.

I have always felt there is a duality regarding our survival instinct and what can only be called a death or destructive instinct. On a lesser level, I would call it a sabotage inclination. I recall times in my life where things were going splendidly, but I would do something self-destructive to ruin it. I know this sound ridiculous, but it is true. I questioned myself repeatedly regarding my self-worth and whether I deserved happiness in my life. I never gave much study to this phenomenon but did come across the work of psychoanalyst Melanie Klein, whose work is well-known in psychology circles.

I find Klein interesting because, according to what I have read about her, she never had any formal academic training. Klein was influenced by the work of Sigmund Freud, and she surmised that humans do have an internal struggle between the life and death instincts that persist throughout our lives. Interestingly, Klein's position was that all suffering is caused by the tension between our creative energy vs. an equally powerful destructive force.

When I read her words, I did not feel so crazy, but it was still disturbing that I had those feelings of destructiveness. I agree with Klein's opinion that life is filled with strife, conflict, challenge, and pain. All humans will face this throughout their lifetime. Klein believes it is productive to find a way to work within the extremes of life and death. I interpret this idea of navigation to mean having the knowledge, experience, and resources to overcome challenges in our lives.

For the suicidal mind, I feel those resources and the support someone needs are absent. Thus, the person feels alone or is tackling the difficulties of life issues on his or her own. This resonates with me because when I was feeling intense depression, I actually felt like I was alone with no one to talk to. I understand now that happiness is not a constant; therefore, it is unrealistic to sustain a constant state of euphoria.

I think it is critical for the suicidal mind to understand this concept. I have never been overly concerned with my happiness. I think it is juvenile and unrealistic to believe that we should constantly walk around in a heightened state of nirvana. It is not that I have given up on happiness; it is simply that it is not a goal of mine to be happy. I experience happy times or moments like everyone else, and I try to stay present in those moments.

I agree with Klein, who says that seeking constant bliss is unrealistic and the root of most of our anxiety and disappointments in life. I happen to agree wholeheartedly with this premise, especially as it relates to the suicidal mind. In addition to obvious depression, a huge part of feeling inadequate is based on where a person is in life vs. where the person thinks he or she should be.

I have startled friends by telling them I go into most situations without any expectations. I try to approach life from a different perspective. I believe it is less likely you will be disappointed in any outcome if you do not have one in mind to begin with.

A good example of this is going on a date. Let's say I consider the night a success if I slept with my date, but the outcome was not what I had planned. We would go out, have a wonderful dinner, see a show, and then go for drinks afterward, laughing and having a great time. If someone asked me about the date later, I would say it sucked because I did not get to have sex with her. That view of the date takes away from the total experience. We had a great time, but because in my mind it had to end with sex, it was a bad date. I think you can come up with other examples in your life where you sought a certain outcome that did not materialize so you considered it a failure.

I think we constantly face an internal struggle. I question myself most when I act out of character or say things that make me wonder who I am as a person. I said hateful things to my ex-wife. Does that mean I am a hateful person because I exhibited hateful behaviors? I realize that I act out of character from time to time, and it upsets me. The internal struggle begins when I falter. I understand I am not going to respond perfectly in every situation. Conflict is inevitable, but I am constantly searching for ways to tolerate conflict and not necessarily seeking nirvana.

I have always felt that awareness is one key to solving any problem. You must be aware that a problem exists in order to address it. I became aware of my destructive gene and tried to understand it.

One of my career mentors used the acronym AUBA to explain how to effectively deal with any business problems. AUBA stands for awareness, understanding, belief, and action. I have discussed awareness and understanding already; the final two steps are the belief that you can effectively change an outcome with your actions. If you do not really believe you can, then you cannot move forward because you will give no effort only a half-hearted effort. Finally, taking action shows you are actually committed to making a change.

I have used AUBA in both my professional and personal life. It is a great way to analyze a situation then sit back and focus on how I will attack problems in my life.

For the suicidal mind, it is critical to be aware there is a crisis. So many times, we do not want to admit our frailties. Since suicide is literally a life and death situation, we must acknowledge and be aware that we are feeling depressed, despondent, or have destructive tendencies. A licensed clinical therapist can help you work through the rest of the AUBA model and formulate a plan toward recovery. I always encourage an individual to seek professional help when dealing with suicidal tendencies.

The journey to self-discovery is a long one. I think back to when I was a child, and first realized that I was my own person. It happened in first grade, and my teacher was sharing our individual portraits with the class. She had us all sit in a circle on the floor, and she pulled out each portrait one at a time. The class then pointed to that student, called out his or her name in unison and then the student had to go to the teacher and collect their portrait. I'm not sure if she purposely presented our pictures in this manner so that we could see that we were individuals, but it had a profound effect on me. It wasn't until that moment that I realized I was an individual. Before that, I thought everyone was the "same" with the same thoughts, ideas and beliefs.

For the first time in my life I was being singled out, recognized for being...me. When I speak of self-discovery I'm referring to an array of characteristics that help form our identities. First, we have our physical features that help identify us to the rest of the world. I like my physical features for the most part, but there are a few that caused me great anxiety when I was younger. My head is very flat in the back, not rounded like my siblings. My brother and sisters constantly teased me about the shape of my head when I was younger, especially if they were angry with me. I was called, "flathead", "iron head", or half a head by my family. It was very hurtful, and I would cry sometimes when they wouldn't relent. People have always commented about my huge, brown eyes too. The comments about my eyes were not always flattering, certainly not when I was younger. Again, I would be teased because they were so huge. Later, my eyes became sort of my calling card with women. They would often comment about how big and beautiful they were, so now my eyes became an asset.

America has a fascination with physical beauty that is increasingly out of balance in my opinion. According to the American Society of Plastic Surgeons (ASPS), Americans spend over $11 billion on plastic surgery each year. That is a staggering number because the bulk of those procedures are to improve aesthetic appearance, and not tied to surgery performed to "correct" damage done by accidents, injuries or birth defects. Physical appearance becomes one of the major ways in which people "identify" themselves. My daughter recently discussed with me the fascination that some of her classmates have with color. She was speaking mainly of her black classmates, who apparently have an obsession with whether a person is light or dark skinned. I can remember this hollow discussion when I was younger too, and it resurfaced again when I read about it in college. The so called, brown paper bag test was used in the early 1900s as a way to categorize black people, and was used to gain admittance into some college fraternities and churches. Zora Neale Hurston, a popular writer, exposed this common practice in some of her essays.

My daughter declared that some of her classmates thought that lighter skinned blacks were superior to dark skinned blacks. Apparently, the light skinned blacks had even started a social circle in which only those with fair skin would be accepted. To my daughter's credit, she distanced herself from one student telling the young girl she could no longer be her friend if she subscribed to such ignorance. I was happy that my daughter took such a hard stance on this issue because it is one that has troubled me for years. There are actually many black adults that promote those same ignorant ideas as her young friends.

Physical attributes can be a way of identifying you, but it simply cannot be the one measure you use to identify who you are. Children are influenced to behave a certain way towards those with disabilities if they are taught to respond to only "beauty" and 'attractiveness" in a positive manner. This is why some children stare or point at people with disabilities because they don't measure up to learned standards of beauty. It pains me to see a child or adult with a disability ridiculed or laughed at by children or adults for that matter.

Surprisingly, there aren't any concrete numbers pertaining to the number of suicides by people with disabilities. In an article published in 1992, Carol J. Gill noted that it was ironic that "so little suicide research has been conducted," on the behalf of people with disabilities since there are so many medical and legal decisions made concerning disability and the management of intentions to die. She was, of course, referring to assisted suicide. The Independent Living (IL) Movement began in the early 1970s to help those with disabilities have a more positive outlook on life, and learn to thrive despite their physical challenges.

My focus here is to try to get people to view others as they are, as human beings before any other classifications.

This includes classifications such as race, gender and sexual orientation. Each of these seemingly benign classifications viewed in the context of modern times have at one time or anther been used to oppress millions historically. It can be argued these classifications continue to do harm particularly in the lesbian, bisexual, gay, transgender (LBGT) communities. The goal is to build the worth and self-esteem of all human beings so they don't succumb to feelings of inferiority, which can inevitably lead to suicidal thoughts.

"Apart from disturbance whose roots are biological, I cannot think of a single psychological problem—from anxiety and depression, to underachievement at school or at work, to fear of intimacy, happiness, or success, to alcohol or drug abuse, to spouse battering or child molestation, to co-dependency and sexual disorders, to passivity and chronic aimlessness, to suicide and crimes of violence—that is not traceable, at least in part, to the problem of deficient self-esteem. Of all the judgments we pass in life, none is as important as the one we pass on ourselves." This excerpt is taken from the phenomenal book, by Nathaniel Braden called *The Six Pillars of Self-Esteem.*

Braden's book is one of the best books I've ever read, and it's one that I have read at the beginning of each year for the past four years keep myself grounded and focused on being me. I've also given this book as a gift to many of my dear friends. I feel it is the seminal work on the subject of self-esteem, and it certainly has great significance on the topic of suicide. I think it is worthwhile to explore some of the ideas that Braden puts forth in his book, which I encourage anyone over the age of 12-years-old to read.

I'm paraphrasing here, so again I'd encourage you to read Braden's book to understand and internalize these concepts fully. He breaks down the six pillars of self-esteem as; the practice of living consciously, the practice of self-acceptance, the practice of self-responsibility, the practice of self-assertiveness, the practice of living purposefully, and finally the practice of personal integrity. Braden has his own views on each of these pillars and how if affect self-esteem.

I'd like to take each pillar and explain why it is important as it relates to suicide or having suicidal tendencies. I think if you read Braden's work, you'll also personalize his ideas, and formulate a solid platform for living your life. First, I would like to explain Braden's point of using the word "practice" in each of these areas. Practice means the discipline of doing something over and over, and not deviating so it becomes a habit over time. Hence, the practice of living consciously is living in the moment no matter what you are doing. I think of this often when I'm playing tennis, or writing jokes. Can I stay in the moment and enjoy playing tennis every minute? Yes! When I'm playing tennis I often touch the strings of my racquet, or gently glide my fingers around the head of the racquet and notice some of the paint chips. I'll look down at the surface of the court and notice how bright and straight the white lines are. I'll squeeze the ball in my hand, noticing the pressure of the ball and the imperfections on the lines.

Practicing consciousness in other areas of my life is interesting too. I love spending time with my daughter, and it's especially important and gratifying to stay in the moment with her. She's banned me from bringing my cell phone into restaurants so that we can have meaningful discussions. She forces me to be in the moment because she doesn't let me off the hook by giving her "yes" or "no" responses. She expects my answers to questions to be detailed and well thought out. Practicing consciousness is trying to have total awareness of who I'm being in any given moment and how I'm acting towards or responding to others. If I remain in the moment and aware, I have fewer and fewer times when I find myself apologizing for an off-handed, rude comment. I am perfectly aware of who I'm talking to, what their sensibilities are, and how my words are affecting them. I've had girlfriends who have commented about how much they like my voice, so of course I was very aware of how my voice sounded in their presence. In fact, I would make sure I had a healthy dose of hot tea and honey to make sure my voice was at its optimal tonality.

"I am what I am," declared Popeye, the popular cartoon character and that pretty much sums up the next pillar; practice of self-acceptance. Popeye's refrain is a reminder to us all to acknowledge our dark side, but to accept the bright side of our being also. The goal here in my opinion is to not be a war with myself. I had to learn that it was quite alright for me to be great or exceptional at something. I could put all my false modesty aside and celebrate being exceptional. How liberating is that? Getting a standing ovation after doing my stand-up act is as liberating as it gets. I have to have a healthy awareness of my impatience or temper in order to stifle those behaviors. If I reject I even have a problem with those behaviors, then I'm starting from a place of weakness.

The next pillar; the practice of self-responsibility is one of my favorites. I think I could write an entire separate chapter on this practice alone, but I'll opt for conciseness here. What could be more important than being responsible for your own life? Before fully understanding the responsibility we have to ourselves, I feel a good starting point is understanding self-responsibility as it relates to early childhood development. I can recall when I was in first grade sitting at one of those small desks that opened from the top. We stored all of our materials like pencils, crayons, scissors and paper inside the desk.

Our teacher explained clearly that the materials in our desk were our responsibility. I think it was the first time I'd heard that word, responsibility. I felt grown up at that moment because even though I was only six-years-old I was entrusted with possessions and expected to protect those items. I began receiving lessons in responsibility at home too. I was responsible for my personal hygiene, bathing, washing my face in the morning and brushing my teeth. I was responsible for making my bed, and keeping the bedroom I shared with my brother clean. Throughout grade school and high school I was responsible for keeping my grades up. I remember there being severe consequences when I didn't.

The biggest lesson in self-responsibility I learned was during my stint in the Army. We had an exceptional drill sergeant during basic training. He was one of the finest men I'd ever met to this day, Drill Sergeant Houghton. Yes, this was over 30 years ago and I still remember his name. Sergeant Houghton was strict, but fair, and he was one of the best teachers I've ever known. He had a sly sense of humor that would come out sporadically if he was explaining a drill or marching orders. I realize he was first and foremost teaching us to be soldiers, but more importantly he was teaching us to be men.

He taught us to take pride in what we were doing whether it was shining our boots, cleaning the barracks, or perfecting our marching drills. He never let any of us "half-ass" it, and I respected him greatly for that. Two stories stand out to me to this day when I think about Sergeant Houghton. The first involved me cutting the dinner line once, and not owning up to it. Sergeant Houghton made me run around the mess hall building until our entire unit finished dining. I then got 5 minutes to eat, and had to help the mess hall staff clean pots and pans. I didn't get back to the barracks until late and still had to finish all my duties in the barracks to prepare for the next day. I was exhausted, but I learned my lesson. To this day, I don't think I've ever cut in line again.

The other story involved our entire unit. Sergeant Houghton took our unit on a 15 mile hike with full gear, backpack weighing about 40 lbs., and our M-16 rifles. We took a water break at about the 10 mile mark, and he allowed us to sit on the grass. Some soldiers starting complaining to Sergeant Houghton about how hot it was and how tired they were. Sergeant Houghton, who was in his early 40s, jumped to his feet and ordered everyone to get up. We were close to a rifle range that had about 50 concrete foxholes in a straight line. He marched us over to the rifle range and ordered us to drop into each foxhole, push ourselves out, and jump into the next...50 times!

After the 50th foxhole, I thought I was going to have a heart attack and die right there on Kentucky soil. To this day, it is the closest I think I have ever been to death. But, I learned a valuable lesson that day, which was no matter how fatigued I thought I was, I always had something in the reserve tank. What I came to learn in the Army is that there are only two results when you embark on any task; go or no-go. That's how many proficiency tests were scored in the military at that time; go or no-go. I loved the simplicity of it because you either completed a task or you didn't. It was that simple.

My idea of self-responsibility was forged during my short four year career in the military. Either I was personally tasked with a job to do or my unit was and there were no "built in" excuses. I either completed the task or I didn't. Success or failure were the only measures I knew. It reminds me of the comedic refrain of the successful comedian Larry the Cable Guy, get 'er done. I've had so many areas of responsibility in my life and I've tried to meet each head on, with no excuses if

I did fail. I began to fully understand the effort and resources I needed to dedicate to certain endeavors in order to be successful. That, coupled with the notion that I hated to fail, propelled me to accomplish many things in my life.

I'm troubled greatly that more people don't take self-responsibility seriously or that it wasn't instilled in them at an early age as it was with me. I think self-responsibility is a cornerstone to having high self-esteem. By fully accepting that we are responsible for our lives, our failures, our successes, our livelihood, our relationships, we take on an ownership which can only strengthen our mental toughness. It is that lack of mental toughness that makes it easier for the suicidal mind to take hold.

The practice of self-assertiveness means taking stock of who we are as individual human beings. This has always been one of the hardest principles for me to master because I have a natural demeanor to fit in, and not cause problems or discord. I learned harsh lessons that if I didn't assert who I was, then I was being complicit in being ignored, or worse being taken advantage of by others. I sometimes feel it's an ongoing battle to be heard, truly heard, and understood. Passivity, in my mind is one of the greatest evils of mankind. I want to be certain that I'm clear that I'm not confusing passivity with humility. I think of humility as a virtue.

Passivity can lead us to places we may never have ventured of our own volition. En mass passivity leads to atrocities such as the holocaust or slavery. Personally, my passivity led to being molested at an early age by a family member. Some people may argue that I was a child and it wasn't my "fault" that I was molested. It was my fault for not speaking up after the fact, not asserting myself. Perhaps my parents didn't teach me to be more assertive that my body was my own and no one had the right to touch me in that way. I'm not sure, but looking back on that incident I wished I was more aware and assertive to defend myself.

As it relates to the suicidal mind, self-assertiveness is essential in not succumbing to negative self-thoughts. I feel you have to constantly declare who you are on a daily basis. I remember watching a motivational video called *Fish*, which is about the workers at the outdoor fish market in Seattle. One the men highlighted in the video talked about having a choice about how he was going to go about his day or who he was going to be that day. I specifically remember him saying, "Who am I being right now?" That has always stuck with me, and I ask myself that question constantly when I interact with others. I want to show self-confidence, and assertiveness, but not in an aggressive manner. Rather, in a respectful manner that says, "I'm being me," to those I encounter.

I speak about living with purpose in chapter 4, so I will move to the sixth pillar of self-esteem, the practice of living with personal integrity. This one is a little tricky for me only because that word, integrity, can mean different things to different people. I will defer to the standard dictionary meaning of the word integrity, which says it's the quality of being honest and having strong moral principles. I like this definition, and I want to explain how this characteristic plays a role in some suicides. The first part of our definition starts with honesty. When I think of honesty, I think in terms of how honest am I being with myself? Part of our internal struggle that I discussed earlier is our honesty with ourselves. Do I have an accurate grasp on who I am as a human being? In that assessment, I have to do an inventory of good and not so good character traits personal to me. I think this is one of the hardest exercises to do if we strip away our egos and are willing to get our hands dirty.

I'm willing to start with my bad traits; moody, defensive, inconsistent, poor follow through, inflexible, selfish, financially challenged, temperamental, and abrasive at times. That hurt just writing those words, and hurt even more reading and reviewing each one. In my mind, those are true, honest faults of mine that I try to keep at bay, and not allow to take over my personality. On the flip side, I get to smile at these positive traits; loyal, generous, intelligent, creative, relaxed, athletic, and eager. If you were to match those good and bad traits against each other you could easily understand why I was at proverbial war with myself.

My integrity or honesty with myself helps me to navigate each of those traits so that I'm not constantly at war with myself. Let's move to the second part of our definition of integrity, which is having strong moral principles. This is an interesting concept to begin with, but even more intriguing since I'm an atheist. I'm often asked where does my moral compass come from if I don't believe in God or follow any religion. Much of my morality came from my parents, who were not church going at all. It could be argued that it does come from religion since I'm almost certain both of them, particularly my mother, have read the bible. Morality to me is built squarely on the premise of if I do this, then this is the consequence.

I tell my daughter repeatedly, that she can do anything she wants, but there is a consequence to everything. I tried to teach her from an early age to focus on consequences of doing something, rather than the act itself. What would happen if I touched this hot stove? I'm going to burn my hand and be in a considerable amount of pain. All of the sudden, the idea of touching a hot stove loses its allure. What if I steal or rob someone? The consequence would be getting arrested, convicted and spending a fair amount of time in jail or prison.

I've been to jail, and visited my brother and nephew in prison. It's not a place I want to be, hence, I don't think I'll be stealing from anyone.

I try to keep my moral bearings to avoid being conflicted. I often confer with friends if I do have a moral dilemma, just to get their feedback and advice on what I should do. This may seem odd considering I'm 51 years old, but I think it's important to seek counsel on big decisions in my life. The practice of personal integrity to me means understanding my moral ground. I don't want to paint this as seeking higher moral ground because there's an inherent danger in that too. I'm speaking of setting a moral compass for my life and following it no matter what temptations or obstacles come my way. Have I faltered in the past? More times than I care to admit here, but that doesn't deter me from staying the course. Moral weakness is just that, weakness in the moment, not fully understanding the consequences of one's actions. I don't think it defines who we are, and it's unfortunate that some people are so unforgiving.

In that moment of taking one's life, I'm certain there is a lack of personal integrity in making that decision. I feel the suicidal person is succumbing or deferring to the "worst' in themselves. They are being deceived into believing they are a fraud of some sort because they haven't been honest about who they are, taking into account good and bad traits. In my moment of darkness and despair, only thoughts of destructive traits were allowed to surface. I struggled to find one positive trait about my life even though I knew several existed. I was not living my personal integrity of knowing I had good and bad traits. Integrity is a cohesion of parts that come together to make the whole. I am a complex human being. That is my truth.

CHAPTER 3

# JOYS OF LIFE

*In the depth of winter, I finally learned that within me there lay an invincible summer.*

—*Albert Camus*

"I don't know what you're shopping for in here, but I'll buy it for you as long as I'm the first to see you in it," I said as she held a pair of barely there panties in her hands.

"That's pretty funny. Who are you?" she asked.

I told her my name and that I was not trying to be funny. She was a pretty Asian woman, small frame with long black hair stretching to the small of her back. She was tan with athletic legs and wore a short black skirt and white blouse.

We continued our conversation, laughing about the merchandise in Victoria's Secret. I learned she was from New

York and visiting Las Vegas to attend a convention. She was shopping before going to dinner with some colleagues.

We chatted about Las Vegas, and I offered her advice on where to take her friends if they decided to go clubbing. She thanked me and proceeded to pick out a few items. I kept my word and purchased a matching bra and panty set and a sheer black robe for her. She insisted I didn't have to pay, but I insisted I did because this was just one part of our deal.

She laughed but took my business card and said she would call me later that night. I kissed her on the cheek and told her to enjoy her dinner. I met up with some friends later that night, and we were club hopping on the strip. We would have a drink or two at one venue and then it was on to the next.

I received a text message about 2 a.m. from an unknown number. It turned out to be Julie, the woman I'd met at Victoria's Secret earlier that day. My eyes widened as I read her message: "I'm at the Bellagio, room 24115. How soon can you get here?"

I tried to wait the required five minutes before I replied, but I couldn't. "I'll be there in twenty minutes."

She texted back that she would see me then.

I told the boys I had to go, no explanation needed or given. I pulled up to the Bellagio valet in nineteen minutes, gave the valet attendant twenty dollars, and asked him to keep my car up front because I didn't know how long I would be there.

I got to Julie's suite, and she opened the door wearing only panties. She had a bottle of red wine opened, and she poured me a glass. We talked briefly about her night out with her friends. She said she had meetings the next day but nothing in the morning, so she was all mine, and I could do whatever I wanted with her.

I have always believed that there are certain seminal moments in life. This was neither, but it was a night I would keep in my mental rolodex for quite some time.

We proceeded to the bathroom to take a shower together. It was a scene right out of one of those cheesy, romantic Lifetime movies.

The shower in her suite was huge, with a marble bench in it. I sat at first and just admired her as she showered. Her body looked flawless under the low lights as the water cascaded down her body. Julie was in her mid-twenties, so her body was firm, and her bottom and breasts had a natural, supple lift.

She eventually turned toward me seductively, and I stood up and kissed her. We continued kissing and making out in the shower for what seemed like an hour but had to be much shorter than that. We eventually made our way to the bed and enjoyed each other until the sun came up.

We parted ways later that morning, and she asked if I could take her to the airport the next day. I agreed.

We got to the airport with plenty of time to spare, and I parked on the upper level of the garage because she wanted to take pictures of the strip from there. I snapped a few pictures of her and then started kissing her. Before I knew what was happening, we were back in the car. I reclined the front seats all the way back, and we had sex in the car on the rooftop of the garage.

Julie thanked me for a great weekend and for driving her to the airport. I had never experienced anything quite like that before. I had one-night stands while performing as a comedian, but this was different. A smile crossed my face as I got back into my car and drove away. It was a feeling of satisfaction and pure joy.

Life is filled with so many pleasures and joys. One way to relish life is to find the joys you love most. Friendships, eating a great meal, traveling, and drinking fine wine are all joys. One joy for me is sex. Yes, I said it: sex.

I realize that sex may not even be in the top ten joys of life for some people, but it is for me. Some may enjoy monogamy, but I am inclined to enjoy the fruits of more than one woman. But I have been in monogamous relationships, and those have been equally satisfying with the right woman.

I have always found sex to be ultimately satisfying. The majority of people enjoy sex with their soul mate, which can be just as satisfying. Either way, the physical act itself is one of the greatest joys of living, in my opinion. There are many ways to connect with another person, but none more intimate than connecting sexually.

The natural pleasure of sex is undeniable to me. Some may try to downplay how critical it is to our overall health and well-being, but I have read so many books and articles that speak of its benefit to our mental and physical health.

It is important that we are responsible in our sex lives for it to be fulfilling. I am familiar with the disturbing statistics surrounding AIDS and other STDs that often come from irresponsible sexual activity. Also, there is a certain maturity needed before engaging in sex. I am advocating sex only for those who are mentally and physically ready to engage in such an intimate act.

When I talk about the joys of sex, I speak from a position of two responsible adults coming together to enjoy one another in an intimate, passionate physical exchange. There are many other ways to show a person you love him or her, but sex trumps them, in my opinion, because sex is so personal. If the sex act is rooted in love, it makes it all that much sweeter. I recall instances where I have actually cried after having sex.

The emotional connection was so great, it truly overwhelmed me.

Before you conclude that I am simply being a slave to my basest instinct, I want to point out sex is not what fuels me. Sex is about passion, and it is best when centered in a deep mental and emotional connection.

If you are fortunate enough, you may have children as a result of your sexual activity. If not, you may join the growing ranks of parents who are adopting or taking in foster children. Either way, taking on the responsibility of raising a child can be one of the most rewarding experiences in life.

I have been fortunate to be a father and have enjoyed a great thirteen-year relationship with my daughter. I think the pure joy in having children stems from the fact that you have an opportunity to aid in their development. In a sense, children are our legacy. My daughter seemingly came into her own around eight or nine years old. She asserted her independence daily in a variety of ways. She no longer needed me to help her bathe or hold her hand when we walked down the street. She began to shape her own identity.

Of course, there is also the not-so-joyous side of raising children. Raising children is an added expense and a full-time job. In most cases, it's a labor of love. But watching your children grow, develop ideas, and formulate their own opinions can be quite joyous.

Even as in infant, children develop rapidly. You likely will see new verbal and physical motor skills every day. It is truly amazing to see a child's growth and resiliency during these formative years. You can even learn from them.

When I divorced, I noticed my daughter handled it extremely well despite the fact she had to live in two homes with slightly different rules. She was forced to adjust to living with my ex-wife's new husband, a person of whom she was not terribly fond. Through it all, she has never faltered. She continues to maintain good grades, and she thrives in several extracurricular activities.

Despite the occasional falls, spills, dog bites, sicknesses, and various parental concerns, I have enjoyed a tremendous boost in energy and awareness and have grown as a person while raising my daughter. She has been the proverbial good kid and therefore an easy child to raise.

It is amazing how quickly I began sounding like my parents. I do not feel that I have been quite as dramatic as my mother or as cruel as my father. I find my parenting to be progressive in that I opt to allow my daughter to fail. I listen to her more than my parents listened to me. I try to give my daughter a voice in our home, and I have allowed that from an early age. She often picks out furniture and pictures, and she has even chosen the color scheme in our home.

I take great pleasure in talking to my daughter. I love chatting with her about the issues of the day. Sometimes I think I have learned more about what is happening in the mind of a thirteen-year-old than I ever wanted to know. She has established her own identity and is quick to share her thoughts on a number of subjects to anyone who will listen.

Another way to add pleasure or joy to your life is to consider a meaningful career. If you work at a job you truly enjoy, then you are fortunate because many of us do not have that luxury. I believe any job that provides for you and your family can add joy to your life. After all, it allows you to do the things that are most important to you.

However, I will acknowledge that working in a job or field that you do not enjoy can have the opposite effect. I worked at a job early in my career that was stressful, and I did not enjoy it. Going to work each day caused me to get terrible bouts of indigestion and even hemorrhoids. Yes, hemorrhoids! It was a true pain in the butt. I recall how my stomach would churn as I drove into work each day.

Eventually, I left that high-paying job to pursue a career as a comedian. It did not make any sense to many of my friends and family because I had just completed three years of law school. I also had passed the bar and began what seemed to be a promising legal career. It was a difficult decision for me. But after weeks and weeks of contemplating the career change, I mustered up the courage to actually leave my law career behind to do what I was really passionate about.

I realize there are many who would see my actions as juvenile and somewhat irresponsible. I knew that I may have been jeopardizing my future, but I followed my heart. I came to the conclusion that happiness was more important. It is much easier to make career changes when you are just starting out; it becomes more difficult when you have responsibilities and people depending on you.

As much as I embraced marriage and eventually being a father, some of my most memorable and joyous times were when I was single. I reveled in hitting the road as a stand-up comedian.

The most interesting thing about this time of my life is that I was the poorest I had been since graduating high school. I traveled from city to city, from one gig after another. Oftentimes, I had to rely on the pay from the previous gig to get me to the next city. It was stressful, but I embraced it all because I was thrilled that I was a working as a professional comedian.

Some gigs were better than others. Surprisingly, the college gigs were the best and paid the most. What was funny about doing college gigs was that no one knew who I was. But for many college campuses, a comedy show was the big thing if there wasn't a sporting event or other function that night. It did not matter if the students had no idea who I was. What was important was that I gained confidence on stage and honed my act.

I think I was most creative during this time of my life. I was writing almost every day. Hysterical bits just seemed to flow. I think college gigs were the best because the kids were open minded. I could really stretch myself with no limitation. I would even adlib much of my show by identifying key groups in the audience, such as the jocks or fraternity and sorority members, and then just ripping on those groups to the delight of the other students. This was a pure joy.

The most rewarding aspect of comedy for me is writing a bit, crafting it by playing with every single word, then taking it to the stage for a reaction. I always gauge how funny a bit is by whether it makes me laugh just reading it. If it is funny on paper, I know I can flesh it out on stage and really make it work. It was as true back then as it is now. I feel my greatest strength at that time was my intellect. I knew I was a great storyteller and that I had stage presence.

Choosing a career is the second most important decision you will ever make in your life. (The first is deciding on a life partner.) There are so many factors to consider when choosing a career. I think high schools need to do a better job of assessing students' abilities and aptitude to guide them on a career path with which they will have the most success. I realize that may not always be easy.

For instance, my story is unusual because the two careers I chose are so different: comedy and law. After all, the two are diametrically opposed.

Career choices are critical because you likely will remain in a particular career for several years. This has changed recently, with many people changing jobs every few years. Today it is rare to find a person who retires after working with only one company. Instead, employees are more like free agents, going to work for the highest bidder as loyalty to one company falls by the wayside. This is another joy in my opinion: having a skill set that allows you the freedom to consider an array of opportunities and accept the one that is best suited for your skills.

Another aspect of being able to choose from a few opportunities is the chance to live in different cities. I have always marveled at Americans' ability to move to any place in the country to pursue their goals. I have been fortunate to have lived in several cities, each with its own charm and identity.

It is curious to me how we take on the character of the city in which we live. My hometown of Providence, Rhode Island, is pretty much a blue-collar area where there was an expectation that you worked hard, raised a family, and died in that city.

I loved the fact that I was raised in Providence because you were forced to be real with people. You could not fake your friendships or what you were about. If you got out of line with someone or ventured to a place where you were perceived as getting stuck up, you were surely going to be put in your place. The refrain might sound something like this: "Get the eff out of here!"

As normal and simple as life seemed back then, suicide was part of reality. I recall when I was a teenager, there was a story in the *Providence Journal* about police captain who took his own life. In his suicide note, he asked a close associate to take care of the police captain's family.

When I think back, two thoughts enter my mind: how much did the stress of the police captain's job play a role in his suicide, and how could he ask another man to take care of his family? Even then, I thought suicide was a selfish act in regards to family and loved ones.

Thank goodness I maintained this opinion throughout my life. It is one reason I decided not to kill myself. Unfortunately for some people, in that critical moment when contemplating suicide, I do not think they consider the lives they will leave behind or the chaos it will cause.

I do not believe the terrible job I had at the time alone would have caused me to commit suicide. Realistically, it did cause a certain amount of depression and anxiety, and it did help me understand the importance of finding a career that would bring me true joy and pleasure.

I encourage everyone to do the same. Find a career that brings you joy and fulfillment. We spend nearly one-third of our lives at work. Therefore, it is important that we choose a job that will bring us a certain amount of joy and a sense of accomplishment.

One of the many questions I ask a woman when I am out on a first date is what she wants her legacy to be. I always get quizzical stares when I ask or am told that no one has ever asked her that question before.

I love the question because it supposes the person will have a legacy, something that others will hold up to show that person's life had meaning. I ask this question because I want to know that the woman I am dating has a purposeful life. I need to know that she is passionate about something.

I contemplated suicide because I felt I did not have a purpose in life, and I did not care about my legacy. Once I made the decision not to go through with it, I set out to find a purpose. Now I am building my legacy daily. Writing this book and the acts of service and lectures on suicide is a part of that purpose.

When I speak of legacy, I do not mean you have to achieve a monumental feat. Rather, I speak of the mark you leave on those closest to you. How will your life be remembered by those closest to you?

Former NFL linebacker Junior Seau committed suicide. To his favor, most of the media portrayed him as a great guy, family man, and philanthropist. I met Seau on two occasions.

A mutual friend introduced Seau to me, and he seemed like a pleasant, humble, and soft-spoken person. I have been around other athletes and celebrities who had huge egos and big entourages, but Seau seemed comfortable, relaxed, and low-key. He was aware of his celebrity but seemed unaffected and treated everyone with respect. He left an undeniable legacy on the football field. He was considered one of the best linebackers in NFL history.

But what is his legacy beyond the football field? A few media personalities were not so kind to Seau, even on the day of his death. Dino Costas, who hosts a nationally syndicated sports radio show, called his act of suicide cowardly and selfish. Others considered his suicide a heroic act, given the spate of concussions suffered by former NFL players. They felt that Seau purposely shot himself in the chest to preserve his brain so it could be studied. Some would argue that the way he died tainted his football legacy.

How do we create a legacy, and what will your legacy be? The best way to answer that is to ask how others will remember you. For the suicidal minds, it may not matter at all how they will be remembered. But it should matter to all of us.

Would it not be great to formulate a plan for your legacy when you consider it will always give you something to strive for, a reason to live and accomplish goals? As I stated before, it does not have to be grand. Your legacy may be that you were a great parent, friend, coach, coworker, volunteer, cook, brother, or sister. Your legacy is what you want to be remembered for, what you pass on to others.

I recall an exercise that an English professor once suggested. It involved the class writing our obituaries. As morbid as that may sound, it was a great exercise. It made us think about how we wanted to be remembered. The idea that someday people will read a few paragraphs about my life fascinated me. Most recently, it might have read something like this: James Bean, casino executive and stand-up comedian, died in his home last night. Bean is survived by his 13-year-old daughter. Bean was employed by Caesars Palace for 10 years, holding various positions in the company most recently as executive casino host. Bean's stand-up comedy career spanned over 20 years and he performed with Dave Chappell, George Wallace and Carrot Top. Bean earned his Juris Doctorate degree and Bachelor's degree from the University of Memphis.

As a young man, you are not really certain of who or where you are in life, so it is chilling to think about. What would your legacy be if you really haven't lived that long? How will people remember you? Will they remember you at all?

I have decided I want to create a more concrete legacy. I am not saying being an executive casino host or a comedian is bad because those are good careers. I am speaking of something stronger when I think of my legacy. What am I going to leave behind? How am I going to be remembered?

I feel I am still writing my story, my legacy, every day. As you consider your own legacy, remember that you are a work in progress, hopefully moving steadily toward a goal. Every day is an opportunity to solidify your legacy. Looking at life in this way gives you a reason to look forward to tomorrow. Tomorrow is a great gift; accept it graciously and use it to build on your life, your legacy.

The good life is a process, not a state of being. To enjoy the good life, we need to do the following: be fully open to experience, live in the present moment, trust ourselves, take responsibility for our choices, and treat ourselves and others with unconditional and positive regard. These are not my words, but the words of humanist Carl Rodgers. He was one of the seminal voices behind moving away from behavioral psychotherapy to a more organic, authentic, free-flowing definition of the human experience. Rodgers' approach is well-regarded in that it removes structure and expectations that come with some behavioral therapy and focuses on an individual's capacity to learn and grow over time. The simple act of being open to new experiences is the key to this approach.

I embrace Rodgers' approach because there is no stated objective or destination for the individual. Being open to each new experience or opportunity and being present in the moment is a great foundation for living a great life.

Abraham Maslow fathered the theory of self-actualization, which states that we all have basic needs that change over time and eventually morph into transcendent ideas of helping others and being altruistic. Rodgers takes a different, more experiential approach to realizing your full potential. I find this approach similar to how I have tried to live my life. Being open to new experiences is one of the key components of Rodgers' approach.

A good counterbalance to feeling despondent or depressed is to be open to new experiences. I call it a counterbalance because depression causes us to focus on internal struggles, and it is focused squarely on the individual. Being open to new experiences broadens our outlook, causing us to look at external forces that may open our minds to new possibilities. This openness must expand to all areas of our lives. I can recall when I was offered new job opportunities with more pay and greater responsibility. Each time I was reluctant to take on the new role, and for a split second I considered not taking the positions at all. My reluctance was totally fear based, and I almost missed out on great opportunities by not looking outside myself.

Another example of new experiences is my dating life. There was a time I would consider dating only Asian women. It was not racism, in my opinion, but rather a preference. I have relaxed my criteria over time, though, and I am more open to dating other women. It was the best choice I could have made. I began meeting exceptional women of different races and entered long-term relationships with a couple of them. Had I remained closed to those possibilities, I would have missed those opportunities.

Rodgers' approach speaks of trusting ourselves and taking responsibility for our choices. I would like to address each of these concepts, starting with taking responsibility for our choices.

I am not sure when this happened in our culture, but Americans play the blame game or find excuses for failure. It is a disturbing trend, particularly when I see more and more adults not taking responsibility for their actions. We have become this culture that needs to find a scapegoat for our failings. It is never the individual's fault, so it seems.

A chilling example of this is the Ronnie Zamora trial that took place in Florida in 1977. Zamora was convicted of killing his elderly neighbor. His controversial defense was that television caused him to commit murder. There are many less egregious examples where people blame others for their lot in life. It is frustrating to me when people do not own up to their choices, decisions, and actions.

I believe it's important to take responsibility for your actions, as our choices dictate our outcomes. If we believe external forces are controlling our lives and we have no choice, why should we get up in the morning? If you believe no matter what you do or whatever is going to happen will happen, you have no control over your life. This thought process can be damning to the suicidal mind. A sense of hopelessness sets in. They feel, "What is the point of living?" I reject this approach and encourage people to take full responsibility for their choices.

Whether we succeed or fail, we can be comforted in the knowledge that we succeeded or faltered by our own actions. What is important to understand is that after a few victories, we begin to trust our instincts more and more. I believe our learning is ongoing, and that you can teach an old dog new tricks. Trusting ourselves means trusting our decisions will benefit us in the long run. It is a process to learn to trust ourselves. Give it time. We make the best decision possible from the information given to us in the moment.

Most people view failure negatively, but I believe it should be viewed positively. Failure can play a major role in a person's decision to commit suicide. I don't consider anything a failure so long as you learn from it. I'm surprised how many people view failure so harshly, as if they are destined to succeed at every endeavor. Supposed failures come in many forms, such as divorce, job loss, or financial loss. I don't think we prepare our children for failure very well. Taking on new challenges means you risk failing. I talk to my daughter about this constantly. I try to explain to her that she should try new things, and put herself into situations where it's a little uncomfortable. I want her to consider outcomes before each endeavor, even if there's a possibility the outcome will be failure.

I have come to realize that failure is one of the greatest ways we can grow in life. Success can be deceiving in some cases because it can lead to a false sense of superiority, causing a person to become lax or lazy. Therefore, failure can allow us to move forward with a renewed vigor and purpose.

I have tried to instill an adventurous and curious spirit in my daughter by encouraging her to try new things and operate outside her comfort zone. I have explained to her that failure is always a possibility. I also have taught her to learn from her failures.

Embrace your failures and own up to them. Failure teaches us what not to do, which is just as important as knowing what to do. The only failure in my eyes is failing to put your hat in the ring, failing to encourage yourself to accept new challenges.

The suicidal mind does not see past today, so there are no challenges. The suicidal mind does not care if tomorrow even comes. This is why it is critical to take on new challenges every day, forcing ourselves to focus outwardly on external goals. It is important to fill our lives with a sense of purpose so we always have something to look forward to. During my crisis, when I was close to taking my life, the thought of tomorrow never resonated with me.

I do not necessarily subscribe to the biblical phrase that an idle mind is the devil's workshop, but I do believe our minds can deceive us into believing we are worthless or colossal failures. Much of our self-worth is contained in how we view ourselves.

There is a natural tendency to compare our lives to the lives of others. There is also a tendency to view our internal thoughts too critically, leading us to doubt our humanity and capability. I once struggled to reconcile my actions to my beliefs. When I acted outside of my character I considered myself a fraud of sorts, putting on a front and hardly living up to an ideal.

The suicidal mind interprets so much information that may be counter to that person's beliefs. I recently discussed with a friend my struggles to have consistent, positive interactions with others. I sought to live above the fray and not succumb to petty differences or ideas. Humans have such a great capacity for generosity, love, and empathy yet equal capacity for hate, destruction, and mayhem.

# CHAPTER 4

# THE CRISIS

*Taking action is how you give your gift and live a life of true service to yourself and others. And that doesn't mean that your life's work has to be something that seems grand and noble. The real key to being of service and living your purpose is simply to do what you love to do— whatever it may be.*

*—Rebecca Fine*

"James, do you know a hospital I can go to because I am afraid I am going to harm myself?"

This was the text message I received from a friend who was depressed because of a financial crisis. The text was surprising for two reasons: I did not know her that well, and she seemed like a person who really had her life together. In my mind, I had no choice but to call in sick at work and drive to her place.

When I arrived, it was obvious she was overwhelmed with stress. I had never seen her without makeup before, which added to her distraught appearance. She struck me as someone who would not think about leaving her home unless she looked her best. She may have even told me that in an earlier conversation. I had only seen her a few times, and she was glammed up each and every time. Her appearance alone told me she was in crisis.

She thanked me for coming over. I suggested she come back to my place after she shared that she feared being alone. She told me she had been thinking long and hard about how she would kill herself: she planned on getting a room at a major hotel on the Las Vegas strip and jumping from its balcony.

I asked her why she felt so despondent, and she told me that her finances were screwed up. She explained that an agreement she had made with a business man from New York to help her get her business off the ground in Las Vegas had fallen through. She further shared that she had already been struggling with her finances and that she was having a difficult time just living day to day.

I told her she was welcome to stay with me and my daughter for as long as she needed. I did not want her to be alone. She had no other friends or family in Las Vegas she felt comfortable turning to.

Just looking at her that day reminded me of when I was in my suicidal state. She had the same hopelessness in her body language. Her face alone expressed her full emotions. She was a personal trainer who normally looked fit and strong, but that day she looked frail in her tiny frame. I feared the worst for her as she told me more and more about her situation and how dire she thought it was.

I pleaded with her to allow me to take her to the hospital, after all, that's why she text me. I wondered at that point was this simply a cry for attention, and not a real crisis. She said she did not have insurance, but I told her I would pay. She said she would think about it. She told me she was somewhat reluctant because of a previous bad experience with a hospital where she had been admitted years earlier for being suicidal. I understood, but I thought going to the hospital would be the best course of action. We ended up not admitting her even though I thought it was the right thing to do. I didn't press the issue because she was already in a fragile state.

She wound up staying at my place for a couple of days. I called in sick the next day to be with her. I did not feel she should be alone. We sat around and watched a lot of bad television and ordered takeout food.

During the course of the day, we talked more about her life and the terrible experiences she had endured since moving to Las Vegas. I asked her once more about going to the hospital, but she refused. I did not want to press the issue.

The next day, at her request, I took her home. I felt strange dropping her off, but she said she was feeling better and thanked me for all I had done. Worried for her, I texted her every few hours. She would reply with "I'm OK." I was on edge whenever she didn't reply immediately because I knew she was still stressed about her financial situation.

Thankfully, her life turned around after her friend agreed to fulfill his promise of funding her business. Regardless, I still worried about her because of how unstable she seemed in those frantic days she had spent with me.

This was the second time within six months that one of my friends had told me she was contemplating killing herself.

The other was a long-time friend who was also experiencing financial woes along with a string of bad luck. She was born and raised in Hawaii. She had shared with me how her childhood was horrific. She was the youngest of a very large family. Her mom was unkind and unsupportive, often telling my friend and her siblings that they would never amount to anything.

My friend owned her own cleaning business and was the single parent of a seventeen-year-old son. The son had recently stolen her car and totaled it, crashing it into a parked car. Now, in addition to her other problems, she did not have transportation to do her job.

I felt bad for her. It seemed she could not get ahead no matter how hard she tried. She had even considered selling drugs during her most desperate times. I really liked her. She was a beautiful woman who was smart and had a good heart. Yet she also had a street side, which reminded me of my sisters. I had helped her out several times over the past few years.

A few years ago for Thanksgiving, I invited her, her son, and several other friends over for dinner and to watch football. Everyone brought food. Both the food and NFL games were great. We really enjoyed the day.

That evening, as we were saying our good-byes, I sensed she wanted to talk to me, but we never had the chance to be alone. About an hour later, I got a phone call from her. She asked if she and her son could stay with me for a few days. She shared that they had been living in her car for about three weeks. I was shocked. I invited her to come back and stay for a few days.

That evening, after they had returned, my daughter and her son retreated to the family room to play video games. This gave us a chance to talk. She shared with me the events of the past few months. She lost her business, and therefore was forced to leave the home she shared with another woman.

I felt terrible as she told me about her childhood experiences and how difficult it was to raise her son alone. She shared with me that when her son was old enough to fend for himself, she planned on killing herself. She felt there was no use in living any longer.

I was surprised by her admission and tried to reassure her that there was always hope. I explained to her that no matter how bad her life may seem, it always has a way of turning around. She said that was nice to hear but, in her case, unlikely. She told me that she had harbored suicidal thoughts for quite some time and was certain she would go through with it when the time was right.

Again, I tried to console her, but she rejected my optimistic view of the future. After about a month, she was able to get back on her feet and got an apartment.

I continued to stay in touch with her. I invited her to basketball and football viewing parties at my home. She came a couple of times, but we mainly communicated through text messages.

One time, she asked to borrow money to pay her rent. Reluctantly, I agreed. I had loaned money to friends in the past, but they rarely paid me back. I explained to her about my past experiences in loaning money, but she assured me that she was not like the others. She assured me she would pay me back as soon as she could. I really did not believe her, but I gave her the money anyway.

Sure enough, she did not pay me back. However, she offered to sleep with me to pay off the debt. I told her I would rather have my money back but, on the other hand, if that was how she wanted to settle the debt, then I was open to it.

We never did have sex, and she never did pay me back. Unfortunately, we had a falling out over the money. During one of our discussions about it, she told me she was ready to kill herself and that she just could not go on any longer. I had heard this from her before, but this time I knew something was different. I felt she meant it.

We were communicating via text messages, and her words were different. Her words seemed dire and more urgent. I got scared. I called my therapist, who directed me to call 911 and report my concerns about my friend.

The conversation with the 911 operator was weird. She was grilling me about why I was calling. She asked a lot of questions, as if it was a prank call. I was frustrated by her reaction.

As I gave the 911 operator all the pertinent information, I got the feeling she did not think it was an emergency. She asked me questions such as, was I with the person? Had she threatened to harm herself before? Did she have a gun or other weapon in the home? Why did I think she was going to harm herself now?

I do not know the protocol for 911 suicide calls, but some of these questions seemed out of line to me. I just wanted the police or ambulance to get to my friend's home.

Finally, the conversation ended with the 911 operator saying she had dispatched officers to my friend's apartment. I then got in my car and raced to her place. When I arrived, she was already engaged in a conversation with the police. The officers seemed satisfied that she was not going to harm herself. She was upset that I had called the police, but she understood why I did it. I hoped this was her last thought or attempt at suicide.

When someone indicates he or she wants to hurt himself or herself or is contemplating suicide, it puts you in a vulnerable position. I feel you must take action, not merely say you took action, and protect yourself from accusations that you did nothing while also protecting or trying to help the person in need.

Some would say I overreacted in this situation, but I feel I did what any reasonable person would have done, given the circumstances. If someone tells you he or she is going to kill himself or herself, you must take action. Call 911 immediately.

I was frazzled by both of these situations because, in my mind, the threat of suicide was real. I do not think I could have done anything differently in either case.

I'm saddened whenever I read news stories where someone commits suicide in response to severe adversity. Such was the case of University of Missouri swimmer Sasha Menu Courey, a Canadian on full scholarship. Menu Courey alleged that she was raped by one or more members of the UM football team. In a report by ESPN's investigative show *Outside the Lines*, it was discovered that the university didn't contact authorities after learning of the incident. Menu Courey, who apparently was already seeking psychiatric treatment, committed suicide a year after the alleged attack. This case is glaring for many reasons, the main one being that Menu Courey and her family felt the university was derelict in its duty to report the alleged rage.

Further, the family said the university distanced itself from giving any assistance or information following Menu Courey's memorial held at the school. While it is always difficult to understand why a person commits suicide, it is apparent when extenuating circumstances contributes to a person's suicidal state. Menu Courey, like victims of bullying, may not have had the mental fortitude to cope with the trauma she endured. This, coupled with the alienation from the university seemingly pushed her over the edge.

## CHAPTER 5

# WHO DEPENDS ON YOU?

*Mistakes are part of the dues that one pays for
a full life.*

*— Sophia Loren*

As pathetic and sad as this sounds, I secretly wanted my ex-wife to miscarry my daughter.

I recall feeling overwhelmed during the time leading up to my daughter's birth. I was making decent money working for Citibank in Las Vegas. We were living in a small, two-bedroom apartment. We would go to birthing classes together but, oddly, I never thought that we would actually see the birth of my daughter.

I have tried to reconcile the feelings I had during that time, but I cannot attribute my less-than-paternal feelings to anything other than fear—fear of the unknown, even though everyone I spoke to said my daughter's birth would be one of the greatest days of my life.

I did not see this as a great event, rather a watershed moment that would change my life forever. Someone would depend on me for everything: food, shelter, clothing, love, and care. I feared I would follow in the footsteps of my father, who abandoned my family when I was about eight-years-old. Would I be that absentee dad? Would I leave and divorce my wife before my daughter was even born?

I lost my focus at work, skipping days and not telling my wife. I reverted to being promiscuous and sought out affairs with a few coworkers. I was reckless during this time, and I didn't care.

When I was a teenager, one way I broke up with a girl was to be such a jerk that ultimately she would break up with me. Fast-forward fifteen years, and I could not believe I was considering employing this strategy to get out of my marriage and avoid being a father to my unborn child.

Months passed and finally the big day arrived. I do not recall ever having such fear and anxiety as I did that mid-September morning in 1999. My ex-wife was experiencing high blood pressure, and the birth was not routine. I was scared. I stayed in the room for my daughter's birth, holding my wife's hand the entire time.

Witnessing a birth is not for the faint of heart. There are what seem to be fountains of blood, and you see the vagina in a state of trauma that remains etched in your mind for years.

Despite the complications, my daughter finally arrived. I don't know whether nurses are trained to say your baby is beautiful, but that was a constant refrain for the next few days from the ones tending to us.

Soler was simply "baby Bean" for a few days because my ex-wife and I could not agree on a name. Finally, we settled on Soler after my ex-wife found the name in a book of baby names. I had never heard of the name before, but it sounded pretty.

My wife did not do well physically after giving birth. She may have suffered from preeclampsia a medical condition characterized by high blood pressure and significant amounts of protein in the urine of expectant mothers. She was also very anxious about our daughter's birth. At one point, she passed out. She needed blood pressure pills and other medication to calm her down. She was out of it for most of the day after delivering Soler. Hours later, she still had not gotten a good look at our baby girl.

I watched as the nurses cleaned up our daughter, removing mucus from her nose and eyes. She was weighed, measured, and then wrapped tightly in a cotton bundle. She was gorgeous. I looked intently at the baby my ex-wife and I had created, and she looked back at me. She did not cry or fuss. I know it sounds ridiculous, but it appeared she was trying to communicate with me through her calmness.

My ex-wife eventually awoke and asked how our daughter was doing. I told her that I knew our daughter was funny because of the curious look she had given me earlier.

Soler has developed an incredible sense of humor since her birth. She understands humor in a way that I never did at her age. When I went trick-or-treating with her when she was three, she had already collected a lot of candy although we had only gone to a few homes. I recall telling her, "Honey, it is nice to share." She replied, "Dad, it is nice to be left alone." It was then that I knew we had another comedian in the family.

My wife was bedridden because of her high blood pressure and could not care for Soler during the first few days after her birth. I was the one who fed and changed her. It is sometimes hard to determine who depends on us beyond obvious family members such as children, parents, siblings, or grandparents. At the time I contemplated suicide, I thought that only my daughter would be affected by my death. She depended on me heavily for her physical, mental, and spiritual needs. If I wasn't around, there would be such a void and who could tell what she might try to do to fill that void.

Then I thought more about others who might be adversely affected by my absence; the list became rather lengthy. I had recently entered into two business contracts, one with the show X Burlesque performing as its featured comedian, and the other with Harrah's Entertainment working in its corporate office. I felt an obligation to finish out my contact with both, especially X Burlesque because the producers had given me my first real chance to perform on the strip. Personally, I knew I owed my mother the greatest debt. She lost two children already, and I felt she would be devastated by my death. She also relied on me financially from time to time.

There were also friends that I knew depended on me. I have always been generous with my time and finances and would lend money to friends in need. I always had a soft spot in my heart for single mothers because I saw my mother's struggle as a single parent first hand. So, I gravitated to dating several single mothers, and even when I broke up with them, I'd still help out financially whenever they asked. I had others in my life that most certainly would be affected by my absence, so they also played a role in me staying alive.

I tried to fill voids in my own life when I suffered from loneliness. I resorted to promiscuous behavior, sleeping with countless women and using pornography. I was absolutely lost. I visualized my funeral and how my daughter might react to my death. I know this is often downplayed because most people have sympathy for anyone who loses their life but maybe not so much for those who commit suicide.

In the end, we all suffer and experience setbacks, devastating losses, and disappointments in our lives. Most of us choose to endure, move on, and face another day, no matter what obstacles we face. I don't know whether a survival instinct is built into our DNA; I just find it unnatural to take your own life, even though I was immersed in that mindset several years ago.

In the classic holiday movie *It's a Wonderful Life*, starring Jimmy Stewart, the main character is given the chance to see how others' lives would have turned out had he never been born. His character is contemplating committing suicide because he believes everything in his life is so bleak.

No matter how bleak things seem, there's always a viable solution but it's not always obvious to the suicidal mind. I wish anyone contemplating committing suicide could see how life continues after their death and, more importantly, how their death affects those closest to them. I believe it's true that suicide is a permanent solution to a temporary problem.

I have experienced incredible friendships over the past ten years. My support system has expanded and strengthened to five friends who would do absolutely anything for me and vice versa. Ironically, one of my friendships blossomed because of a suicide.

A friend's husband committed suicide and several of her closest friends rallied around her, offering her support in various ways. Everyone did their best to help her cope with the tragedy. She and I had always enjoyed deep, insightful conversations. Our discussions got deeper as we tried to make sense of her tragic loss.

She once asked me, "What is the meaning of life?" Without even thinking about it, I blurted out that it's to live your life. She laughed at the simplicity of my answer.

We spent many long nights just talking about life, its meaning, and if life even had a purpose. We didn't debate the topic, it was more exploratory. Her focus was more on the careers we choose and how we enter in and out of other people's lives. She was devastated by her loss, and I did my best to comfort her and offer her hope about the future.

Suicides are devastating because the survivors are left feeling guilty, helpless, and despondent, always wondering what they could have done or said to prevent it from happening. My friend dwelled on her perceived role in her husband's suicide for months, uncertain about what she could have done differently. She focused on the signs she missed regarding her husband's behavior in the months leading up to his death. How could she have missed the signs of depression? Was she too busy to see the signs? Did she play a role in his decision by not being available to talk? No doubt she will ponder these and other unanswered questions for the rest of her life. This is why suicide is never final—at least not for the living.

When I think about life, I think about how much of it is built around relationships and how we cultivate those relationships depending on their importance to us. People who commit suicide fail to acknowledge their relationships and how important and viable they are, especially if they involve a spouse or a child. In the case of a spouse, depending on the length of the relationship, there are many memories that combine to make both parties vested in the bond. What I mean is, there is a history, and that history is the mutual bond between the two people.

I have been in several long-term romantic relationships, and when each ended, there was a natural sadness and sense of loss. I felt vulnerable, afraid, uncertain, betrayed, and abandoned. These emotions came on quickly and intensely.

I tried to move on with my life and function as best I could. However, with a few of my relationships, it was hard to let go. I would rehash moments where I behaved badly or was unsupportive. I would think about how I could have acted differently. I contemplated what I could have said differently. It was always frustrating trying to reconcile how two people can be so in love and supportive one moment and in just a few days or weeks, they can reach a point of no return. In some cases, they end up hating each other.

Now consider a relationship that ends when one party commits suicide. The sense of loss would be devastating; it certainly was for my friend. The hardest thing about losing a partner to suicide is the feeling of helplessness and being left with the question of why your partner made such a terrible choice. The finality of suicide alone would be shocking to anyone.

Sometimes discord leads to domestic violence, as in the case of former Kansas City Chiefs linebacker Jovan Belcher, who killed his girlfriend, Kasandra Perkins, and then later turned the gun on himself. The highly publicized murder-suicide was shocking for many reasons, especially because it left the couple's three-month-old daughter without parents. Ironically, the Kansas City Chiefs organization had tried to provide counseling for the pair weeks before the tragedy.

One image etched into my mind about this incident is the press conference conducted by Belcher's teammate, quarterback Brady Quinn. He gave an eloquent plea for everyone to be present for their friends and have conversations that go beyond superficial and trivial matters.

Belcher's actions were reprehensible. This is why so many consider the act of suicide to be cowardly and selfish: you leave behind people you love to deal with the wreckage.

No one can go inside the mind of a suicidal person other than assuming there is some kind of mental anguish causing the person to end his or her life. So many thoughts are streaming through that person's mind.

Most people consider the consequences of their actions before doing anything that drastic. We do this when we move to a new city, buy a car, or take a trip. So how can suicidal people ignore the consequences of their actions—or do they? In my case, I did. Unfortunately, some people are not strong enough to do this or they are so distraught they can't see the consequences.

This supports the idea that suicide is a selfish act. If someone commits suicide knowing how it will devastate those closest to him or her, then it is selfish. The problem with suicide for me lies in the fact that when someone commits suicide, he or she doesn't suffer any consequences or, more accurately, isn't held accountable for them. Yes, in death, the person who commits suicide is vilified, but this is as useless as giving posthumous awards to athletes or entertainers. I am not saying that the person should be punished since he or she now is gone. Rather, I am suggesting that suicide is the only act we can commit and not have to answer to anyone about it.

We owe our loved ones respect, compassion, and care. In life, we are held to a certain standard to provide support and love. We show this by being present in their lives and keeping our commitments to them. When you bring children into this world, you have committed to putting a roof over their heads, getting them up for school in the morning, or driving them to soccer practice. When you get married or live with someone, you commit to following through on date night, taking care

## | WHEN THE HUMOR IS GONE |

of your partner when he or she is sick, and making sure the bills get paid. Depending on your level of commitment and the depth of your relationships, people depend on you every day, perhaps in ways you have never considered. We honor our loved ones through service and with our lives.

Of course, there is another side to suffering through life as a sacrifice for others: when the people in your life act as your tormentors. I think of all the children who deal with parents who are unsupportive at best and mentally or physically abusive at worst. I cannot imagine how it is for a child to live with parents who are abusive and negligent.

Some children also face brutal hazing or beatings at the hands of bullies. Often they face this abuse alone because schools don't do enough to protect them. The recent spate of teen suicides is alarming. Many of these suicidal children were harassed for being different, mainly based on sexual orientation. In California, three teenage boys were charged with sexually assaulting a classmate while she was passed out, then posting photos of the alleged attack on the Internet. A week later, 15-year-old Audrie Pott committed suicide. Another is the case of Staten Island teen Amanda Cummings, who killed herself because of relentless bullying by some students at her school. These are just two examples of teens taking their lives in response to awful events that happened to both of them.

The point I am trying to make is that for many suicidal minds, the prospect of leaving behind loved ones is lost because of the intense pressure to alleviate a terrible situation, all because the person is being bullied or tormented daily. Most often, the tormentors have no idea that their actions are literally driving a person to end his or her life.

There is a call to action by parents and extended family to embrace teenagers no matter their sexual orientation and reassure them that home is a safe place. Our criminal justice system has to be revamped so that hate crimes are prosecuted more aggressively, and that convictions carry lengthy sentences.

I can only imagine the psychological pressure placed on children who are not only dealing with internal struggles based on their sexuality but also external hazing by classmates who have labeled them misfits based on their sexual orientation. It saddens me that our society is not more protective in light of highly publicized murders, such as Matthew Sheppard's. There are teenagers who are aware of his plight, and they are opting to take their own lives rather than face the possibility of being the victim of a hate crime like he was.

Parents have a responsibility to be involved in their children's lives. They are responsible for what their children may do to others. Think about it: prejudice is a learned trait, not inherent.

I hope that everyone has someone to live for, but I realize that isn't always the case. I have taken specific actions in my life to make sure that my daughter, mom, sisters, and closest friends know I care about them. I have found, at least with my daughter, the most effective means of showing love and concern is by looking directly into her eyes when we talk. This may seem like a small gesture, but it is effective.

I do not call my mom or sisters as much as I should. However, when I do, I make a conscious effort to move beyond the mundane questions of who, what, and where, and instead focus more on how they are feeling.

I must approach each of my sisters differently because of their varying personalities. With time, I have found a way to build a meaningful connection with each of them.

I think men are the hardest to connect with, but once a bond is formed, it can be a lifelong relationship. I have two such friendships with men that I have cultivated over several years. Because we sometimes are caught up in the alpha-male syndrome, there is a natural barrier that must be broken. I have broken that barrier by being humble, supportive, and nonthreatening to my male friends. This allows ideas and thoughts to flow freely with little or no judgment.

The key to bonding with anyone and building a relationship that could deter someone from acting on suicidal thoughts is finding out where his or her interests lie and taking a genuine interest in what is important to him or her. If a person builds a network of people who have a stake in that person's goals, I think it makes it that much harder for the person to commit suicide when things get tough.

# CHAPTER 6

# IF YOU WERE NOT HERE

*I say you ought to write out ten outrageous goals that are bigger than you because your life isn't meaningful or important unless you're on purpose about something way bigger than you are.*

—Mark Victor Hansen

So you are dead—now what?

I have often wondered in those few dark moments before a person actually commits suicide if he or she realizes that tomorrow is another day; it is inevitable, and it is coming.

I can recall even as a kid visualizing my own funeral. Who would show up? What would be said? How soon would I be forgotten? Picturing the funeral was funny in some regards. I wondered how I would be dressed. Who would decide what I wore? Who even knew what my favorite suit, tie, or shirt was? I have gone to so many funerals and seen good makeup jobs and horrendous ones. Would the mortician make me look like a movie star or more like a corpse?

When I was a kid and thought about my death, I just thought people would come to a big church, a few words would be spoken, and then people would go to my mom's house and eat potato salad and ham. Funerals have always fascinated me because it was always about mourning instead of celebrating the person's life.

I grew up as a Catholic, so ceremony was important. To me, the Catholic church had a hierarchy of services, which I would rank top to bottom as Christmas, Easter, weddings, funerals, and finally normal Sunday services.

Funerals were interesting to me. I understood the loss and the fact that everyone grieves differently, but I always felt that I was forced to feel sad the whole day after attending a funeral.

My grandfather's funeral was the first that I ever attended, and it was a beautiful service. He lived well into his eighties, yet I did feel a loss. His funeral was well attended, and I cried during almost the entire service.

I think it would be beneficial for anyone who is contemplating suicide to understand they will be mourned by a number of people. When a person commits suicide, his or her life ends, but life goes on for everyone else—a continuum. I don't believe anyone with a suicidal mind is able to fully comprehend all the people they will leave behind.

I once read a book by David Deida called *The Way to the Superior Man*, where the author talked about life and how it never stops; there is always something more ahead of us. It ends, of course, for the person taking his or her own life, but the person must understand that life continues for those left behind. A person thinking of taking his or her own life needs to understand the effect the act will have on everyone with whom that person is close.

At the time I was contemplating suicide, my boss gave me some great advice when I told him I was getting a divorce. He brought me into his office and showed me his calendar. On it were several travel dates for him and his wife. He said part of their bond and how they managed to stay together was the trips they would take. He said when his wife looked at the calendar, she always had something to look forward to. This made so much sense to me. I wish I had established such a plan in my own marriage.

I think of life much in the same way, we need things to look forward to. I have always believed you need a reason to get up in the morning.

My main reason for getting up in the morning is my daughter. I have a great relationship with her. I have been fortunate to see her mature and grow into a beautiful young woman. I have enjoyed the talks we have had or, as she likes to point out, all the laughter.

Without my knowledge, my daughter read the manuscript for this book. I had saved the document on my computer, which is not password protected. When she saw the title, I suppose she was curious. I could not figure out why my daughter used to ask me on more than one occasion whether I liked my life. I thought it was an interesting question coming from an eleven year old, but now I understood the context of the question.

I had to spend a great deal of time reassuring my daughter that I no longer had suicidal thoughts. I told her I had not harbored those thoughts in several years, and that I did in fact love my life. In a way, I felt like a failure as a parent because my daughter now knows that at one point her father considered killing himself. This was sobering for me.

I imagine what it would be like if my mother or father had suicidal thoughts. Would they have shared their thoughts with me at any age? At eleven, my daughter was already mature for her age. Regardless, I feel the knowledge of her dad's suicidal tendencies was too much for her young mind, no matter how mature.

The reality is there is no turning back the hands of time. She already knows, so I can only hope she takes the lesson from this devastating time in my life and uses it to help others.

The following two text messages are one my daughter sent to me and one I sent to her when I found out she had read the manuscript on my computer. We had discussed her reading it the night before. I wanted to reassure her that I was going to be fine:

"Thanks, Dad. Sorry I did not reply earlier. My phone was off and in my locker. I am really glad you did not do it. We would not have all the fun times together—like when we watch *Hoarders* or the first part of *The 40-Year-Old Virgin*. Anyway, I am really glad to still have you here with me. Love ya, Junie."

"Soler, I love you very much, and I love my life, too. I'm glad we talked about the book last night. I was going through a bad time back then, but things have changed. I'm in a better place, and I promise to be with you for a very long time."

Junie was my nickname growing up, and my daughter enjoys calling me that. I started crying after reading her text.

I quickly thought about how negatively my daughter's life would have been impacted had I followed through with committing suicide and was overwhelmed. I now realize she would have endured so much pain and possibly been lost without my guidance and presence. The psychological scar would have been on her for years, and she may have decided to end her own life at the slightest hint of stress. I felt ashamed at that moment for even considering ending my life.

My daughter was six-years-old when I contemplated suicide. In the seven years after that bleak moment in time, we have shared a number of great experiences, including two special vacations.

A friend suggested that I take my daughter to Costa Rica for vacation one year. We had a wonderful time exploring part of the country. I had befriended two women on Facebook, and both were exceptionally cordial to us the entire time we were there. They took us to local restaurants, beaches, and sight-seeing. My daughter got to meet local children and play in their neighborhoods. She didn't speak Spanish, and the Costa Rican children didn't speak English, but they played and enjoyed each other despite the language barrier.

Two years after the Costa Rica trip, we traveled to Auckland, New Zealand. I had met a young Chinese lady in Las Vegas who lived in New Zealand. We e-mailed each other periodically and when our vacation came up that year, I decided to travel there. By this time, my ex-wife had already remarried, and my daughter was not fond of her new stepfather. It was a difficult transition for her.

The New Zealand trip solidified relationship with my daughter because we had great discussions about how she was feeling about my divorce and her mother's subsequent remarriage. My daughter told me she felt she'd betrayed me because her mother would not allow her to tell me she had remarried. I did not learn of her marriage until a year later.

My daughter exhibited a level of maturity I did not expect from her at nine years old. We explored New Zealand's countryside, hitting almost all the tourist attractions along the way: beaches, caves, ocean views, farms, and parks. New

Zealand was one of the most beautiful places we had ever visited. To this day, my daughter speaks fondly of our trip there.

Traveling with anyone can be a bonding experience, and traveling with my daughter allowed her and me to bond in ways I could never anticipate. Even our travel within the United States has given us memories for years to come. She has seen some of the great US cities, including Seattle, Memphis, Los Angeles, Miami, San Diego, and Washington, DC. Each trip has its own unique story for her.

Life does continue, and we have the opportunity to realize our dreams and goals if we continue living. There is such finality to suicide; much more than just in the literal sense. Suicide is an interruption to life for everyone involved.

What better reason do we have to live than to love another human being? This is an interesting, complex question because I am certain that some suicides have been the result of romances gone wrong. I have never been in love in the true sense of the word. I have adored women and had great affection for them, but I have never loved a woman unconditionally. I did not even love my wife in a romantic sense. I married her because I thought she would be a good mother.

I have read so many books about love and romance and what it means to be consumed with another person. There is a side of me that believes this is the best thing we can hope for in our life. On the other hand, I see the danger in sharing your feelings with another person.

According to the National Institute of Justice statistics for murder-suicides continue to climb in America. In fact, the U.S. has three times as many murder suicides as Canada, and eight times more than Great Britain. Most murder suicides are domestic in nature or involve some element of a scorned lover. Despite these dire statistics, I still hold out hope that I will fall in love and settle down. I have always thought that having another person pledge to love you unconditionally is one of the great joys of life. I have never had that feeling of completeness, and my quest to find my other half has been a lifelong pursuit. Finding and being in love is a great reason to be alive.

Having a reason to get up in the morning is critical to feeling alive. Your life must have a purpose. Without purpose, life is like the movie *Groundhog Day* starring Bill Murray. Murray's character goes through the same day over and over again until he finally "gets it right."

I can see where the redundancy of our lives would adversely affect our desire to live. What exactly are we living for if each day is almost identical to the previous day and the previous day to that? We have a responsibility to ourselves to shake things up, to make each day a portrait in itself. It is a blank canvas, and we are the artists applying the brush strokes to make it amazing.

# CHAPTER 7

# LEAVING A VOID

*The first hundred years are the hardest.*

*—William Mizner*

I sometimes purposely think about life without some of my family members and trusted friends. It is an exercise that I have done for several years to help me evaluate my relationships and how I would be affected if they did not exist.

I begin with the relationships that are most important to me. I think of the void I would have in my life if I did not have my daughter. As a parent, there are times when you cannot remember when you didn't have children. With the rash of teen suicides, it is not far-fetched to think I could lose my daughter to suicide. The thought that anything could happen to her disturbs me. One of my daughter's middle school classmates was killed by a drunk driver. I cannot imagine the pain that her parents had to endure.

I think about all the activities I do with my daughter now: playing tennis, going to the movies, taking trips to the bookstore, or going on vacation. Just to think of doing all those activities without her is depressing.

I take this so seriously, I am specific when I think of my life without her. How would her room look? How soon would I discard her things—or would I? Some people make a shrine when they lose someone. Would I do that for her?

I think about how the basic things would change in our home, from cooking to doing the dishes. How would my spending habits change? Would I buy the same items from the grocery store? My daughter's favorite drink, cereal, or snack food? Everything would be different.

When my daughter rides with me in my car, she sits in the back seat because she says it is more comfortable. I think it is because she does not trust my driving. I like our drives together because we talk freely about a variety of subjects or focus on the news of the day. This is where many of our conversations begin. I always glance in the rearview mirror to look at my daughter as we talk. When she is not present, I purposely look in the mirror and glance at an empty seat. My point in doing this exercise is to fully understand how different my life would be without her.

Tragically, there are parents who live what I only imagine. Somewhere in the world today, a parent lost a child to disease, a car accident, or suicide. They are faced with the reality that their child will not be coming home. The Trayvon Martin tragedy highlights this point. He went to the store for Skittles and iced tea, a fateful decision that left his parents without their youngest son. They are forever faced with that void.

## | WHEN THE HUMOR IS GONE |

As I have stated before, I think a suicidal mind never considers the void that will be left behind. That is why most people consider suicide a selfish act. The void left in the aftermath of a suicide is expansive and goes far beyond the mere absence of the person taking his or her life. There are so many things that survivors must consider. There are financial repercussions, mental anguish and, of course, the all-encompassing question of why?

Unless you had intimate knowledge of the person who committed suicide or he or she left a detailed note, everyone who had a relationship with that person is left wondering why? I have discussed this many times with my friend whose husband committed suicide. It was especially painful for her when she has to relive the anguish whenever one of his friends calls who is unaware that he took his own life. This is stressful on her, and you can feel the pain as she explains the circumstances surrounding his death over and over again.

The aftermath of suicide reverberates for years, as the survivors cope with guilt that often turns into anger. Many times, survivors are left in the unenviable position of reviewing the last few weeks or months of a person's life, trying to find any clues about why their loved one would commit suicide. This was an excruciating exercise for my friend and painful to watch.

What I find interesting about death is how life goes on after we are gone. I used to joke with my friends that if we were to die or be fired from our job, the company we work for would continue on as usual. Our contribution to our work, no matter how large, is only a blip on the radar. Sure, in the case of a death, there would be an obligatory memo sent out by the company and maybe even a memorial for the person, but beyond that, it would be business as usual. This is why I never boast or get too full of myself, no matter what position I hold in an organization.

Suicide, on the other hand, is a special case for employers. Organizations must tread lightly; otherwise, the company may appear to canonize a person who took his or her own life.

I believe this was the case with Junior Seau's suicide. A public memorial was held, with many former teammates and friends attending. Some spoke and hailed Seau as a hero. Some even called him courageous and a great man. Others shuddered at those words. They saw Seau's act as cowardly. Yes, his athletic prowess and achievement on the football field remain unchallenged, but his off-the-field decision to end his life was not necessarily deemed courageous.

Tomorrow will come whether or not we are here. And I assure you, those days when you are having the most difficult time, when the entire universe seems to be conspiring against you, will pass.

When I was in my own suicidal state, I could not see that. I could not see beyond that day—the day I was going to end my life. I mark the anniversary of that day on my calendar, just to remind me of all the good days that have happened since. It is amazing how much can happen in an eight-year span. I have changed jobs three times and always for the better. With each job, my responsibility and salary increased. I have seen my daughter grow from a little girl into a beautiful young woman. I have made new friends, and solidified relationships with old friends. I moved into my dream house, which I share with my daughter.

Suicide is the ultimate silencer of dreams. It can prevent greatness from ever materializing or coming to fruition. I asked a good friend to read and give me feedback on the introduction to this book. She said what my daughter said, which is she was happy I did not make that fateful decision. She was happy we met and, if I were not alive, I would not have enhanced her life as I did.

Suicide reminds me of the movie title *Girl, Interrupted*. Perhaps a better title would have been *Life, Interrupted*. You have a life that is filled with all the highs and lows we all experience, but during a low point, the person decides to end it all. Again, it is hard to reconcile suicidal actions in the wake of knowing that life has many vicissitudes.

I hearken back to that common refrain that suicide is a permanent solution to a temporary problem. Life is filled with so many disappointments and devastating events. I have learned to put all of my problems into perspective by considering other people's problems. I think comparing your troubles to others may not be the most effective method of putting events into context, but it does offer some perspective.

I can think of so many devastating events that may bring someone to consider suicide: the death of a loved one, divorce, financial ruin, physical impairment. The psychological strain alone is enough to make even the most resilient of us vulnerable to suicidal thoughts.

I will use divorce as an example since I have some experience with it. Divorce is essentially one person telling you that you are not worthy or, more specifically, that you are not worthy to be with them. The devastation of that lies in the fact that the person making this declaration was once your greatest supporter and ally. It stands to reason that if the person who knows me better than anyone else rejects me, why wouldn't everyone reject me? Again, although the person who loved you the most at one time is making this declaration, it does not mean you are not worthy of living.

I realize that, in the grand scheme of things, my life is not, nor has been, as rough as millions of others. I do not have to worry about where my next meal is coming from, nor have I ever. I do not have to worry about having a home to live in, nor have I ever. If I were to put my everyday life in place of those far less fortunate, one could argue what am I complaining about?

This is not to diminish the psychological pain that accompanies a divorce, job loss, or other life-changing events but simply to put those events into context. When you think about it, are those events so devastating that you must end your life because of it? My answer is a definitive no. The fact is, unless someone is facing severe mental or physical pain, he or she needs to endure it until it subsides—and it will subside. The old adage that "this too shall pass" is true—it usually does.

I cannot help but think of the regret a person who committed suicide would have if he or she could see the next day. I personally know how hard it is to get past that moment when you want to end your life. But, when in that moment of despair, try to remember the old adage, "There will always be a brighter day." It really is true. There is always something worth living for.

The void that is left is more than just the absence of the person who committed suicide. It is the void of what was to come, the possibility of what that person's life held or the potential to enhance the lives of others. The void is even greater when you consider the potential legacy a person could have built had their life not been interrupted.

There's a great line from the movie *Apocalypse Now*. Captain Willard is given his assignment to end Colonel Kurtz's command with extreme prejudice. I have always remembered the statement, "When a suicide is complete, that life ends with extreme prejudice. It ends with such suddenness and volatility, it sucks up everyone in its wake like a high-powered vacuum."

## CHAPTER 8

# THE PURPOSE OF LIFE

*Oftentimes the test of courage becomes rather to live than to die.*

*—Vittorio Alfieri*

"James, if this shit was easy, then everyone would be doing it," one of my law professors said to me when I was contemplating dropping out during my second year of law school.

My sister had been murdered that year. I had feared the worst because, when I was home over Thanksgiving weekend, I did not see my sister Debbie the entire time. If ever I had an excuse to wash out of law school, this was it.

But I attended my sister's funeral and returned to campus. I still had a few midterm exams to complete. I took my law books home, but don't recall opening them while I was there.

Law school, like my military training, was making a man out of me. The objective was to graduate, as Malcolm X would say, "by any means necessary." My grades in law school were less than stellar; I maintained a C+ average. This was encouraging on one hand because I wasn't flunking out but depressing in that I was trying my hardest and only getting Cs. In many ways, I owe it to my friend Rick Komistek, who was also my roommate at the time, for even going to law school.

Rick is one of the smartest people I've ever met, and he currently is a professor at the University of Tennessee. He said I could debate any topic with anyone, and that I'd be a great lawyer. I was dismissive of his comments at first, but then I reconsidered and actually took the LSAT and scored well. The University of Memphis offered me a full scholarship to law school, which I accepted.

I was at a crossroads of sorts, kind of drifting and not knowing exactly what I would do after getting my undergrad degree. I was working and making decent money, but I did not love my job. It was a weird existence because I was doing just that: existing. I had no mantra, no true purpose.

Law school gave me every challenge I could ever imagine. I wasn't the smartest student there; I had to work exceptionally hard just to keep up. One of my law professors told me that unless I could explain each case to a six-year-old that I didn't truly understand it and all its nuances.

I was forced to read case law four, five, even 10 times before I mastered it. Law school wasn't like my undergraduate classes where you could never read the textbook and assigned material but still skate by. In law school, every professor called on you and asked pointed questions about the cases and assigned material. My last name begins with B, so I was in the front row if we were seated by name. I preferred to sit in the front even in classes where there wasn't assigned seating. Since I was one of only four black students in my law class, I got called on a lot—more than most other students.

It forced me to be prepared for each class. I had to read and be prepared to be successful. I read and prepared with myopic focus and determination. In my estate and property classes, the professors would always call on me if there were racial implications to the case, such as unenforceable or restrictive covenants. These were interesting cases where someone would buy property and one of the conditions of the contract or ownership was that it could never be sold a black man. I had three law classes each day and was sure to get called on at least once a day in one of those classes, so I had to be prepared all the time.

I recall sitting in class on my first day of law school and crying. I was that overwhelmed, not because of the material, but because I was this black kid from the ghetto of Providence, Rhode Island, and there I was in law school. I could not believe my good fortune. So from my first day in law school, I was preparing for my last day and walking across the stage with a law diploma in hand. My meandering ship now had a rudder.

For the next three years, I stayed the course through two years of celibacy, my sister's murder, and my brother's death from complications of AIDS. I did not waiver from my purpose to see my law studies through. When I did graduate and walked across that stage, it was one of the biggest turning points in my life. It showed me what dedication, motivation, and purpose could bring to my life.

What is the purpose of life? I think the question is an exercise in futility. When friends have posed that question to me, I have simply stated that the purpose of life is to live your life. I was not trying to be flippant by giving that answer; it is genuinely how I feel about the question.

I don't oppose anyone trying to find meaning or purpose in their life. However, in the pursuit of an answer to that question, I feel some people are not truly living their lives. I feel this is one critical reason that many people commit suicide. In their search to find meaning and purpose, they are often left disillusioned by the possibility that there is no true purpose to life.

I liken trying to find purpose in life to a person seeking true love. That person goes through life with a definite composite of what true love is. He or she considers appearance, drive, ambition, career, height, weight, skin color, voice, and even the type of car his or her true love should drive. Consequently, that person passes by hundreds of eligible candidates, never giving them another thought, because these people don't fit the unreasonable criteria.

I have never allowed an ideal to supersede reality. That is not to say I do not have goals or dreams; I dream as much as the next person. However, I have never sacrificed imagined joy for real joy that I can experience right now.

I think of the countless people in the dating pool who are adamant about waiting for the right one or not settling for just anyone. Again, I am surprised that more people do not see the futility in this approach to finding a lover or lifelong partner. You are not settling if you give someone you would not otherwise consider as soul-mate material a chance. On the contrary, you are opening yourself up and considering the possibility that others outside your stated criteria could fulfill your romantic desires.

This also fits into the idea that "all the good ones are taken." It would be like going to a movie that is sold out, and you opt to see another film. You find you are perfectly content with the second film. In fact, it may be more enjoyable than the one you originally wanted to see.

When a person commits suicide, often it is because he or she failed to find purpose in life or a reason for living. My challenge to the suicidal mind is to ask yourself, "Do I need a reason for living?" Is not the fact that you are alive a viable reason for living your life?

I once read a book called *Why Your Life Sucks* by John Lester. In it, Lester challenges readers to look at all the stresses, trials, and tribulations associated with their life. He then makes this startling assertion: in the majority of cases, we create our own problems. I initially was defensive when I read this statement because I thought it was one of the most insensitive passages I had ever read. However, upon reflection, I had to agree with him.

As I thought more about my life and my own greed, ambition, and poor decisions, it became clear that I was responsible for the majority of the frustrations I faced. This was not easy for me to admit because I am not the type of person who claims to be a victim.

The difficult part for me was taking full responsibility for the heartaches in my life. I began to think about my divorce and how my actions played a role in that process. I thought about the times people took advantage of me. When I look back, I realize my own selfishness, greed, or personal agenda caused me to be duped. Had I exercised due diligence and restraint, I probably could have avoided 90 percent of the turmoil and drama in my life.

At my lowest point, I began to reflect on all the bad decisions thus far. I was alone, despondent, divorced, and desperate with seemingly no one to talk to. Having thought about it, I began to understand that I bore much of the blame for my situation.

Now I can see how I was unbearable to live with during that time. I looked calm on the outside, but inside I was about to erupt. My ex-wife caught the brunt of my anger and frustration, as did my daughter. I use to lash out at my ex-wife for practically no reason or, as she used to say, "Lay into her at the slightest infraction." I'm not proud of this period of my life, but it was important that I acknowledge how difficult I was to live with then.

In part, the shame I felt about myself led me to being suicidal. In my mind, I had failed my family, and I was failing financially and professionally. In my mind I had become a failure. Eventually, I was alone and depressed, and the chasm was getting wider with each passing day. The chasm was the divide between where I thought I should be and where I actually was in my life. In my mind, I was living a lie because I was not living the life I envisioned for myself. I also struggled internally with obvious contradiction between how others saw me, and what I knew to be true about me.

I think others saw me as a pretty solid person based on my charming demeanor. I was like a man coated in Teflon, nothing negative ever stuck to me. I had an ease and unflappability about me. I could be sullen, but I never displayed that in public. My public persona was one of competence, confidence and discipline. Internally, I felt I was lacking in all of those areas. Perhaps I did have a high opinion of myself that wasn't grounded in reality. If I had the ability to compare my standing with others, I would have been able to conclude that I was in a better place than most professionally, and financially.

I visited a therapist who reassured me that I was fine. Given my age, education, and current financial situation, I was right where I should be in life. But the therapist's words fell on deaf ears.

I still felt that I was an underachiever, a common person, a failure. The pressure to have the life that I had envisioned was clouding my judgment. I felt I should have achieved so much more at this point in my life. My situation reminded me of a song by the Talking Heads, "Days Gone By," where part of the refrain is, "Where is my beautiful wife? Where is my beautiful home?"

My ambition was working against me. Everything seemed to be crashing down around me because, in my mind, I had nothing. Even more mentally damaging was that the future seemed quite bleak. I realize now that I was doing this to myself. I clouded my mind with the wrong expectations of where I should be in life and what I had become: a failure.

When I think about what's happening in the mind of a suicidal person, so many emotions come to the surface. I am not sure people really appreciate or understand the psychological strain that the suicidal mind endures during times of duress. It is overwhelming.

To truly understand how a person could even consider taking his or her life, you would have to place yourself inside that person's mind. Think of a time when you were at your absolute lowest. Now multiply that by one hundred, then take away any support system you have. Now consider that this current psychological state you are in is permanent. In fact, you are convinced there is no relief in sight. Now you are getting close to understanding how the suicidal mind operates. Ending it all is the only viable option to a person who is suicidal.

For the suicidal mind, purpose, reason, ideals, and zeal for life are replaced by an apocalyptic view. You convince yourself it is all going to end—if not for the world, certainly for you.

Everything becomes clouded. Minor setbacks are magnified to the thousandth degree. Even the most normal natural desires we have in life, such as food, shelter, sex, personal interaction, and basic survival are absent.

Consider the magnitude of feeling that it is all right that today is your last day on earth. Losing the desire to partake of life's simplest pleasures is tragic. That is why I feel it is more important to enjoy life than pursue the reason or purpose for being here. When challenges and strife become your main focus, it becomes more difficult to enjoy the simple things that used to bring you so much joy.

I'm proud of the fact I have been able to pursue things that bring me pleasure. I would not necessarily say it is a hedonistic pursuit. I try to compartmentalize my life. I do my best to do what I enjoy the most on a daily basis.

I took up tennis a few years ago. I found that I really enjoy it, so I now play three or four times a week. It is a social sport, and I am constantly meeting new people to play against. A good friend recently took up salsa dancing, and she invited me to a free lesson. It was amazing. Afterward, I decided to sign up for more lessons.

Another simple pleasure has been spending time with my daughter, such as watching movies together. It does not matter whether we go to the local theater or simply watch them at home. It has become a ritual with us, even though my modus operand is to fall asleep during the loudest and most action-filled scenes.

I also have found that I enjoy debating various topics with my friends. It is a pleasure having spirited conversations about topics such as sports, politics, love, relationships, or parenting.

Food became one of my delights when I started working in the casino industry. Las Vegas has transformed into one of the epicenters of culinary delights over the past decade.

Before, I never really considered food to be enjoyable beyond it filling me up and energizing me by fueling my body. It was after my divorce that I found myself trying just about every restaurant in Las Vegas.

When I began serial dating, every time I dated a new girl, I tried a new restaurant. I still had my "closing" restaurants, too. There were two or three I would frequent that I knew would guarantee me sex when I took a date there. This is when I learned how food and wine served the purpose of being an aphrodisiac.

This was a simple pleasure I discovered that made my life worth living. I enjoyed being on a date with a beautiful woman, dining at a great restaurant, and being filled with the anticipation of how the night might end.

This brings me to women—another one of my simple pleasures. I have always embraced the sexual tension or energy that exists between men and women. No matter where I am—working, shopping, jogging or running errands—I live for those moments when I pass a woman and feel her energy. This happens to me regardless of a woman's age or attractiveness. In fact, it is more powerful with older women. Perhaps this is because they embrace their sexual energy. In any case, this enjoyment is a simple one.

Passing a woman, I can make eye contact with her and, in that instant, there is an unspoken agreement that, given the right opportunity, I could take her as my lover. This may sound egotistical or nonsensical, but I assure you that I have lived those moments most of my adult life. I have truly enjoyed this type of exchange thousands of times.

However, I do not want you to think I disrespect women in any way. I have always looked at women with great admiration. Women are subjected to inequality seemingly at every turn. So when I have the opportunity to give that look of acceptance, of understanding empathy, I do it without hesitation. Again, it is an unspoken exchange in most cases, but in those rare moments when it instantly becomes a romantic pursuit, I embrace it fully.

I have often wondered whether something similar happens when a woman sees an attractive man. Do they receive what I term "masculine energy"? For me, it is a joy to receive a woman in this way, if only for a brief, fleeting moment.

Psychoanalyst Erich Fromm speaks about the ideal productive personality, where an individual seeks and finds legitimate solutions to life through flexibility, learning, and sociability. I agree with Fromm that we should strive to be rational, and approach and respond to the world with an open mind. We should always be willing to change our beliefs based on new evidence that may run counter to our established beliefs.

One of those established beliefs may be how you view yourself. When we accept a negative view of ourselves, there is a danger that those views become permanent, so we stay in a state of depression. That is why it is important to challenge your beliefs and ideals on a regular basis. This exercise is not to change your view of life but rather to offer a new way of looking at yourself and the world, especially in a depressed state of mind.

Fromm finds that we should aim to become one with the world. It is not at all about assimilation; in fact, it can be quite the opposite. Fromm refers to such a person as "the man without a mask." By becoming one with the world, a person can escape the loneliness that comes with separation.

It takes courage to live transparently. I have learned to do this as I have gotten older. I allow myself to be more open with my thoughts, ideas, and beliefs. For a long time, I didn't want to tell anyone that I was an atheist for fear of being judged and ostracized. Having read extensively about this topic, I have formulated arguments in favor of atheism. I did not do this to win debates; I just wanted to articulate why I believe what I believe. More and more, I began feeling comfortable discussing this important aspect of my life. I was no longer afraid to show friends exactly who I was.

I strongly believe we all want to be a part of something: a group, a cause, a movement. It can be exhilarating. The danger of assimilating into a group is that, many times, the individual dies in the process. Fromm's view is that we all should retain our individuality because therein lies the strength of the group. We can strive to become unique individuals, according to Fromm, and still have a yearning to join a group and have unity with others.

There is a danger in conformity and assimilation when you join a group. The individual becomes voiceless and faceless in the pursuit to blend into the group. This is a dangerous proposition, according to Fromm. I agree because, through conformity, no matter how dynamic and unique, the individual dies a slow death over time. The individual essentially becomes one with the group and a shell of what he once was.

I also agree with Fromm on the topic of developing a strong sense of self through learning. Discovering our own ideas and abilities is the key to true self-awareness. The suicidal mind is distorted because it never seeks or acknowledges the greatness and uniqueness of the individual. I am not speaking of individual greatness in a narcissistic or delusional sense, rather in the sense of understanding and embracing our uniqueness.

I am convinced that the person contemplating suicide does not realize he or she offers value through his or her uniqueness. It is unfortunate that instead of feeling empowered knowing that they are unique, suicidal people feel they have no power. They feel they are not special and have nothing to offer friends, family, or society. The irony of is, one reason I came to write this book is because my friends embraced my uniqueness and were interested in how I differentiated myself from others as far as my thoughts, beliefs, and ideas. My ideas were not so much original in my mind. I think I viewed things from a different perspective, and I expressed those ideas passionately.

Fromm maintains that we can find wholeness and meaning through discovering our individuality. By following our own ideas, creativity, and passions, we forge confidence and conviction in our lives. Our conviction does not have to come from religious dogma that originated centuries ago. We can develop new purpose and conviction based on our experiences and simply live out those convictions without worrying whether they are accepted. This is a freeing of the mind that I feel is beneficial for everyone. To free the mind, you must take away the stigma of measuring up to someone else's ideals.

The suicidal mind is fraught with distorted images, illusions of what a person should be. This is because a suicidal person feels he or she does not measure up to what he or she perceives society expects of them. This can be true in one or more areas of life (e.g., career, looks, education, financial status, sexual prowess). If you lose a lover, you feel distraught that you will never find another person to love you. If you lose your job, you feel you will never get a job opportunity as good as the one you had. If you are experiencing financial difficulties, you feel you will never regain financial stability and you will always be broke.

The trouble is the suicidal mind creates a false sense of reality. That person has convinced himself or herself that the situation will never change. We know this to be false because life is full of change; it is the only constant we know.

We have a duty to ourselves to embrace our individuality and constantly work to improve ourselves through self-discovery. Forget what society expects of you. We grow exponentially by seeking new challenges, defining ourselves, and embracing our personal uniqueness. We need to be bold, learn to love greatly, and understand our place in the world. Our goal in life is to achieve a level of confidence and maturity that is underlined by self-discovery. This enlightenment can then be used to contribute to the collective and not alienate ourselves through self-absorption.

# CHAPTER 9

# LONGEVITY

*Why do we do anything? Are we our actions,
or something more?*

*—Anonymous*

The following is a passage from Dr. Martin Luther King, Jr.: "Like anybody, I would like to live a long life. Longevity has its place. But I am not concerned about that now. I just want to do God's will. And He's allowed me to go up to the mountain. And I have looked over, and I have seen the Promised Land. I may not get there with you, but I want you to know tonight that we as a people will get to the Promised Land."

Those words have always resonated with me. Dr. King was speaking of his own mortality, knowing in his heart that his days were probably numbered because he had already received several death threats. I cannot imagine the type of stress and pressure he was under during the turmoil of the Civil Rights Movement of the 1960s. I like that he talked about longevity and how it has its place, but that it is not ordained for everyone.

When I think of longevity, I think about one of my goals or measures of success: having grandchildren. I envision myself as a grandfather sitting with my grandchildren, recounting all the crazy stories of my life. I picture myself schooling them about life. I do not want to be that older person who is out of touch with today's youth. It takes effort to stay connected with young minds.

Some of the best years of my life were teaching at a small high school in Maryland. I coached the boys' basketball and football teams. Just being around kids keeps you young, listening to their fears and helping them navigate those difficult high school years.

It is important for adults to listen to kids and empathize with their plight. The issues children face today are far greater in scope than when I was I kid. I see it firsthand with my daughter. We talk about the various issues of the day, speaking freely and openly about everything, including sex. I never had a conversation with my parents about sex. I want my daughter to feel that she can talk to me about anything.

I have open discussions with my daughter every day. We talk about whatever issues come up, whether it is about drugs, abortion, religious rights, or human rights. The media gives us plenty of topics to talk about. We discussed the school shooting in Newtown, Connecticut, and it was interesting to hear my daughter's ideas of how to improve school safety. We even discuss the authenticity or honesty of the media.

My point is that I try diligently to connect with my daughter on a real level, an honest level. I hope to continue this with my grandchildren, who will invariably ask me about the "good-ole" days."

I find a certain comfort in having turned fifty. While many would say fifty is not that old, I disagree. Fifty is old as hell—or at least I feel it is. I measure my age by listing events that have happened in my lifetime. The computer, internet, cell phone, and microwave were all invented during my lifetime. I remember the big cell phones that looked like the old combat radios, complete with the long extending antennas. Our kids cannot imagine a world without cell phones and computers.

There were other seemingly unthinkable milestones that happened during my lifetime. A man walked on the moon in 1969. The Berlin Wall came down in the 1989, and the world watched as Russian Communism fell apart in 1991. I cried as I watched Barack Obama win the presidential election in 2008—the first black man to become president of the United States of America.

My point is longevity has its perks. I think of all that has happened in my lifetime, and it amazes me. I recall how excited I was to see the turn of the millennium. I whipped out a calculator when I was a kid and calculated how old I would be in the year 2000 (thirty-seven). I thought about how old that was, and I wondered what I would be doing and where I would be living.

It seemed so far away at the time and when it finally came, it was like a blur. I would often think of Prince's hit song "1999," which was released in the early 1980s. But then, just like that, it was actually 1999. When I consider longevity, I sometimes think about the friends and family who are no longer here and all that they have missed.

Longevity does have its place. I see life as a timeline that is different for each of us. I think of the events in my life that I can recall vividly, such as Dr. King's assassination, my daughter's birth, the first time I had sex, the LAPD's pursuit of O.J. Simpson in a white Ford Bronco, the night Howard Cosell reported that John Lennon was murdered.

I also recall the event that changed America forever: the September 11 attacks. I marvel at my ability to recall those events as if they were happening right now.

I now realize that the suicidal mind does not think of future events. Instead, the suicidal mind focuses squarely on what is happening in the moment. It does not see beyond the present, which is dangerous.

I recall being in that state of mind and not being able to imagine a tomorrow. I could not envision waking up, showering, watching television, or starting my car and going to work. I could not see past the razor blades and pills that were in front of me.

It was not until I could gather myself together and come to my senses that I could see my situation clearly. Suddenly, I could see a future with my daughter. I could see a life of happiness for myself and hope for a brighter tomorrow.

I started to recount what a great life I had lived up to that point. I realized how much I had accomplished, and that there was so much more in front of me. I wanted to write more jokes. I wanted to enjoy more women. I wanted to eat more juicy steaks. I wanted to travel with my daughter. I wanted to write this book. Even if you live to be one hundred years old, that would not be a long time in the grand scheme of things.

So why would anyone want to cut their already-short life even shorter? My message to anyone contemplating suicide is simply this: no matter how dire or severe your situation may seem, it will pass. Your problems are only temporary. Time has a way of resolving all issues.

I associate this with going to the dentist for a cleaning and knowing you will be in pain for the next hour or so. You won't be in pain the entire day unless your dentist is terrible. He will finish and give you some tips on how to floss more effectively so he does not have to do as much during your next trip. My point is you know you will be in the chair for about an hour and then it will be over. The decision to see the dentist for a cleaning would not be easy if you knew you would be in that chair the entire day.

When we are going through a life crisis, it seems as though it will never end. Even if you manage to find a respite while in this state, often the solution is less than appealing.

"This too shall pass" is a familiar refrain. It is true; whatever strife or obstacles we face, time becomes our friend. That doesn't mean there won't be lingering effects. Sometimes that is inevitable. But the storm, the crisis will pass in due time.

It may be difficult for the suicidal mind to understand this, but time becomes your ally. It is amazing when I look back on all the times I was at a low point—especially when I was preparing to take my own life. Those difficulties became faint memories over time. Sometimes I can barely remember what the crisis was because time passed so quickly.

I have always been fond of photography, taking photos and then looking at them. I still like looking at family photos or pictures of world events. When I look at a personal photo, I consider it a snapshot, both figuratively and literally. Figuratively, it represents an entire moment in time captured in a fraction of a second. Perhaps it is a snapshot of me with my daughter or of me performing on stage. It may not tell the whole story, but I can fill in the rest. A photograph says, "I was here. This is what I was doing, and this is why." It gives you something to think about. It offers you a glimpse at the life of someone who lived.

Every photograph, every memory is a brushstroke of our life. And when we pass, the painting of our life is complete, perhaps for the world to see. Longevity allows the canvas to be filled, eventually to be appreciated by those who were touched by your life.

Committing suicide is like having an artist put the brush down. He stops painting mid-stroke, and now the canvass is unfinished. Anyone who views the painting cannot make out what the artist was trying to portray. There is no feeling or emotion surrounding it. This is an example of why longevity has its place.

The longer we are here, the longer we have to positively affect the lives of others. We have time to realize our goals, look back on our accomplishments, and have the satisfaction of knowing we built a legacy.

CHAPTER 10

# THE ONES I KNEW

*The conscience of death accompanies us since childhood, as conscience of the absolute destruction of the only precious treasure of ours: our I.*

—*E. Morin*

On May 2, 2005, Francisco Vega, a ten-year air force veteran, hung himself inside his garage. Cisco, as everyone at the theater called him, moonlighted as a doorman at the V Theater where I performed in a production show.

Cisco was funny and fun to be around. He always had a mischievous grin plastered on his oval-shaped baby face. Cisco and I, along with others from the theater, would occasionally go out for a drink after work. The drinking and boisterous talk usually took place at one of the many Las Vegas strip clubs.

Cisco and I hung out one night with two women from his unit in the Air Force. As ridiculous as it sounds, we entered a popular lesbian hangout located inside the hotel where we worked with the hopes of getting laid. Cisco and I laughed uncontrollably at our desperation, which led us to gawking for hours at the hottest lesbians on the strip. It was quite amusing to watch two 6'3" brothers in the middle of the dance floor totally oblivious to anyone in the club. Invisible horny men—it sounds like a movie title.

Cisco always struck me as a person who had his life together, sans the usual demons we all possess. When I say demons, some may refer to them as vices or anything that might be considered a character flaw. Certainly drugs or alcohol abuse would fall into this category. Other addictive behavior like gambling could be considered a personal demon too. Cisco's demon was alcohol abuse. In addition to working at the theater, he also had a solid career with the air force. We always had pleasant, superficial conversations. The topics of our conversations were mainly sports, women, or cars.

Cisco was married, though you would never know it by his actions. He hung out, drank, and frequently ran with the bartenders from work. He talked of his love for his autistic son and the challenges he and his wife had raising him.

I always joked that working at the theater was like the movie *Groundhog Day*. Much like the show I work in presently, I was the nightly featured comedian. Almost every day I would come in and say the exact same things to the theater employees: "What's up? How are you? What's happening? It sure is slow tonight. Hey baby. What's up, bro? You look good tonight. I like your hair. Busy tonight, isn't it? Can you get my friends in? Can I get a drink? Give me a pound, bro. Hi pretty, how you doing', girl?"

This type of bantering went on day after day for more than two years. The funny thing is I did not know the names of half of the people who worked there.

After a time, you begin regarding the people you work with as family members because of the frequency of your contact with them. Being with Cisco and the others at the theater nightly, I formed a relationship with them by default. What was interesting was that I did not even know if these people liked me. My interaction with them was on such a superficial level it became difficult to discern who was a fan and who despised me.

Cisco, on the other hand, was a little different. Even though I knew him on the same superficial level as others in the theater, I always felt a certain warmth toward him. I felt he respected me and my act.

It was not unusual for Cisco to give me suggestions on how to tighten up my act. He liked that I never asked the doormen to deal with hecklers. I always handled it from the stage, and he respected me for that. We had a mutual respect for each other.

I knew he was in the military and understood that he took on this gig to make extra money for his family. It saddened me that he had to work so many hours. I knew that every morning he would have to get up at 5 a.m. after having worked until just after midnight on most days. I had been in the military myself twenty years earlier, and I remembered how most of the men with families held down other jobs to make ends meet. It is shameful that those protecting our liberties are paid so little. I do not know if fatigue contributed to Cisco's fateful decision, but it certainly could not have helped.

I attended Cisco's memorial service in a local Las Vegas mortuary. Though ultimately well attended, the crowd was sparse when I arrived early. It was one of those sweltering Vegas afternoons: it was early May, but the temperature was already 95 degrees.

Standing outside the chapel, I noticed a few servicemen from the Air Force and several employees from the V Theater. I signed the guest book and entered the chapel where his body was resting. I approached the altar and knelt down by his body. I was the only person in the chapel at that time, and for some reason it actually felt good. This was my chance to communicate with him one last time.

Cisco did not look at all like himself. He was darker in color and looked smaller lying in the casket. He was 6'3" and weighed at least 250 lbs. Yet in the casket, he looked like a frail, skinny person. He no longer had the oval baby face; instead it was narrow, and his cheeks had sunken in. It was the first time I had noticed that the tip of one of his fingers was missing. I do not know if it was from his death or if it had been that way for a while.

As I knelt down beside the casket, I began to weep. Still alone with him in the chapel, I sobbed uncontrollably for what seemed like ten minutes. I looked down at his body, realizing that I would never see him alive again. I would never again see his tremendous smile or shake his large, soft hands. Cisco would never again pull one of his notorious pranks or look at a beautiful woman in his flirtatious way. He would never again take tickets from a patron or carry trays back to the kitchen. But the saddest of all was that he would never hug his son again. This was final; he would never do anything again.

I finally stopped crying and regained my composure. Next, my mood turned hateful, almost violent. Anger took over as I looked at his face again. "You bastard!" I thought to myself.

"Who the hell do you think you are to kill yourself? Why did you do this and leave this horror for us to deal with? Do you know how many people you just hurt by doing this? How could you? I never told you this, but I cared for you. I loved you for the human being you were. You were a cool guy and my friend, so why did you have to do this?"

I began to calm myself as I carried on with the mental conversation. "If you had to do this over, you would do it differently, wouldn't you? What were you thinking? What is wrong with you? You have a child. You can't kill yourself when you have a child. Are you sick? Are you demented? What the fuck is up with you, Cisco? You are wrong for what you did."

At this point, it seemed like all the air had escaped from my lungs. I was getting dizzy as I knelt in front of the casket. I began to think, "What are you doing going off on this corpse that's lying in front of you?"

I knew what I was thinking was wrong, but I could not let it go. Cisco's death was the third suicide that had affected my life, after my little brother assigned to me through the Big Brothers/Big Sisters program in Memphis and an associate I worked with at the hotel.

Timothy, or "Little Man," as my little brother's family fondly called him, was a precocious little black child assigned to me by the Big Brothers/Big Sisters organization. I joined Big Brothers/Big Sisters because my older brother had a Big Brother when we were growing up. He was really nice and generous to both my brother and I. Though I don't recall his name, I do remember he was tall white man who had just graduated college and was beginning his career.

Technically, he was supposed to take only my brother on outings, but he allowed me to tag along on several occasions. He took my brother and me to our first NFL game to watch the then-named Boston Patriots. We sat in the nosebleed section, but it did not matter because we were seeing players that we had seen before only on television. I felt fortunate to join my brother and his big brother on these outings.

Timothy became my Little Brother during my sophomore year at the University of Memphis. I had settled in as a student and did not have a heavy academic load that year. I had started working, so I had a little cash to spend on Timothy, though the agency cautioned me against spoiling him.

Timothy had a little brother, who also had a Big Brother assigned to him. We would sometimes do things as a group, or his Big Brother and I would alternate and take both boys on outings.

Timothy was a lot of fun to be with. We would play basketball, go to the movies, or sometimes go to the park to just sit and talk. I remember taking both boys to wrestling matches at the old Mid-South Coliseum. I would also take the boys to the University of Memphis basketball games. This was a big deal at the time because Memphis was very good, regularly appearing in the top twenty basketball rankings.

My relationship with Timothy was great. He shared a lot of his personal life with me and, after a while, we began to consider each other family. I recall the time he invited me to Thanksgiving dinner. I initially declined, explaining that Thanksgiving was a time for him to spend with his family. He said I was family. His sincere words made me tear up.

I mentored Timothy for nearly three years. Unfortunately, when I graduated from college, I started working on a regular basis. I didn't have as much free time, so we got together more sporadically, usually once or twice a month when before it had been every week.

I will never forget the disturbing phone call I received from Big Brothers/Big Sisters to inform me Timothy had been shot. I asked what hospital he was taken to so I could go see him.

The coordinator said it was a fatal wound, and Timothy did not survive. She expressed her sorrow, and I hung up the phone. I collapsed backward into my chair, covered my eyes, and began crying uncontrollably.

My thoughts turned to his mother. I pulled myself together, then got up and closed the door to my office. I went back to my chair, sat down, and picked up the phone to dial his mother. When she answered, she was hysterical. I did my best to offer my condolences. At first, I was at a loss for words. Somehow, under the circumstances, I managed to say I was sorry and told her to please let me know if there was anything I could do. She said she would call me in a day or two with the funeral details.

I sat at my desk numb, tears streaming down my face. I was in a state of shock and disbelief. I would never play basketball with him again or see his infectious smile. I had this knot in the pit of my stomach as I tried to reconcile what had just happened.

Over the next couple of days, I assembled more information on how Timothy died. Apparently, he had been involved in a botched robbery. The police pursued him all the way to his home. Timothy got there first, ran inside, and hid under a bed with a gun in his hand. I was told that when the police entered his mother's home, the gun discharged and the bullet struck him in the head. It was never made clear whether Timothy's death was accidental or a suicide. However, given the circumstances, it is likely the fatal wound was self-inflicted.

Timothy's death affected me deeply. I felt as though I had failed him. I questioned whether I had failed to instill decency and integrity in him. Did I discuss doing all the right things in the right way and the importance of not running afoul of the law? I was sure I had, so why were we trying to deal with this tragedy?

Timothy's mom did not have any insurance and no way to pay for his funeral. I gave her the money to pay for the memorial and burial; I wanted nothing in return.

Timothy's funeral was nearly unbearable for me. Lying in the casket, he looked like the little boy I had first come to mentor. This was partly because, even though he was seventeen when he died, he was only 5'3."

Timothy's death was one of the saddest moments in my life. I was devastated. I began to regret not being a more positive influence in his life. I was hurt that he had chosen to engage in the illegal activity that had played a major role in his death.

I don't know why I tortured myself by thinking of his last moments. I could not stop thinking about him under that bed with a gun pointed to his head. I tried to imagine what was going through his mind in that last crucial moment. His death would haunt me for years, but it was not the last time I would face someone's suicide.

A colleague from the hotel ended her life abruptly a few years ago. I remember the last day I saw Holly: the day before her suicide. She was her usual funny, affable self. Holly would joke and flirt with me all the time. She was a pretty woman with a nice smile. Holly reminded me of the actress Ellen Barkin, blonde hair with an athletic body. Holly always appeared to be in good spirits. The last day I saw her was no exception.

She left work around 7 p.m. and popped her head into the casino host office, affording me what would turn out to be one last look at her patented, goofy smile. She was one of the few people who could always make me smile and laugh. There was no sign that this would be the last time I would see her beautiful face. Just a few weeks earlier, she and another coworker came to see my show at the Flamingo. I was as shocked as anyone when I learned of her death.

Holly was only thirty-six when she died. I recall all the people who attended her memorial service and how sad they were. I sat with her coworkers and wept throughout the memorial.

Holly and I were not acquainted well enough for me to know what she may have been dealing with in her life. I now regret this. I realize I cannot be fully immersed in the lives of everyone I know, but I think it is important to have substantive interactions with people.

Since Holly's death, I have tried to be more engaging and have meaningful conversations with all of my coworkers. It can sometimes be difficult because people at work tend to be guarded. There is only so much information they are willing to disclose, but I do not allow that to keep me from trying.

Since those deaths and my own attempted suicide, I have read several books and articles on the subject. I have done a tremendous amount of soul searching to try to understand why a person would take his or her life. No one really knows what goes on in a person's head that leads them down the path to suicide.

I wish I had all the answers, but I don't. One reason I am writing this book is to make everyone aware of how powerfully everyone I have met thus far has influenced my life. This is a personal account of what I have experienced with suicide. I trust that those mentioned understand that I am writing this book with one motive in mind: I want my thoughts and ideas to serve as a cautionary tale.

The only truth that I have come to realize in my fifty-plus years on this earth is that you must try to positively influence those around you. The people you come into contact with everyday need their buckets filled. I think that we all start out the day with our buckets filled with water to use an analogy. Well, throughout the day others take our water, and by the end of the day we may be left with nothing. I like to help replenish people's proverbial buckets with positive energy, encouragement, and acts of service. Everyone has hopes, dreams, and goals, and you could be the person who leads them to pursue their goals and dreams. I thought I had influenced some people in my life who ultimately committed suicide but apparently not enough.

I cried uncontrollably when I wrote the suicide note to my family. I was truly prepared to go through with it. I was despondent about so many things in my life. I was unhappy about my failed marriage and, in my mind, I was not doing well in either of my professional endeavors: working at the hotel during the day and performing as a stand-up comedian at night. Everything seemed to have come to a head, and I was not prepared to go on with my life. I was ashamed of making the decision to kill myself, but I honestly did not see any other way out. I had become extremely tired and frustrated all the time.

I would get up at 8 a.m. and go to work as a customer service director for Caesars Entertainment at its corporate office and perform as a comedian at 10:00 p.m. almost every night. It was the same revolving door day after day. The difference between me and most others who work two jobs is that I was very sick. I was suicidal. I liked doing both jobs; however, both were extremely taxing on my mind and body. I felt as though I had no energy. I was drained emotionally and physically.

Most of my friends could sense something was wrong but did not inquire beyond the superficial discussions of work and dating. I wanted to tell someone about my depression but who? The closest I came was during a telephone conversation with my older sister Sheila.

My sister was intuitive and real, as they say. She could always sense when things were not right with me. She told me I sounded depressed, and I blurted out, "I am!" She asked if I was seeing a therapist. I lied and said yes. The truth was I had stopped seeing my therapist months earlier. I just did not feel comfortable talking about my depression to anyone. At the time, I had been divorced for about a year. I never had great conversations with my ex-wife, and she had recently thrust herself into Christianity. Since I reject all propositions of a higher power, I did not want to hear her preach to me.

I felt like I was on my own, as if I was on a deserted island, but in reality, I was surrounded by people most of the time because of my jobs.

My day usually had many highs and lows. My job at Caesars Entertainment was interesting. I later worked directly at the hotel as the customer service director. I came into contact with so many guests and hotel associates, I sometimes felt like the mayor of the hotel. Performing in a show on the strip used to be fun, but I was so distraught that it, too, became a job with no joy. I know that this showed through in some of my performances. I felt like I was an angry man on stage trying to make people laugh. Thinking back on it now, it was quite bizarre.

During this time, I contemplated suicide almost daily. Then, at night, I would go on stage, trying to make a room full of total strangers laugh. I wish I could have been like my idol, Richard Pryor. Pryor would have gone right on stage and talked about wanting to kill himself and how he was going to do it. I haven't been able to take my personal life and make it funny on stage. Instead, I rely on one-liners, fictitious stories, and exaggerations. I always thought my life would make a great book or movie. It has everything: sex, violence, death, pain, and family strife. It would make the true American story.

One of the biggest frustrations I experienced during this time was trying to figure out how I got there. I was a quiet, sensitive child and smart by everyone's account. I cried when I could not go to school. I often think, how square and nerdy was that?

I was the middle child of divorced parents who never really divorced. As a result, when my father died, my mother received his Social Security, military and other pensions. It did not matter that they had not been together for more than thirty years.

It was poetic justice when you consider my father had never paid my mother one dime of child support. Fortunately, my sister Sheila and I had made peace with my father months before his death.

Prior to my father's death, Sheila learned that she was not my father's biological daughter; her biological father had died two years after my father passed away. Sheila had always felt she was not my father's daughter by birth. My father confirmed this revelation while he was in the hospital. He thought he was going to die, so it was a death-bed confession. However, he lived ten more months.

My mother was furious that my father told Sheila that he was not her father. To her credit, Sheila forgave my father for not taking this secret to his grave. In a strange way, this brought them even closer. She provided him with comfort and constant companionship in the final months leading up to his death.

Given the fact that he had been hospitalized earlier, my father's death did not come as a surprise. I was so sure that his death was imminent that I jumped on a plane to Fort

Lauderdale to be with him on New Year's Eve. I stayed about a week to help get his affairs in order.

When I arrived, I was shocked at the conditions under which he was living. In fact, to say I was upset was an understatement. He appeared to have little or no support from family members living in the same town. I stayed at his house while he was in the hospital and spent most of my time cleaning the place. I could not believe how filthy it was. Supposedly, he had a maid, but it appeared she only cleaned once a year.

I actually met her and recall how proud she was when she declared to me that she was my father's housekeeper and had been for two years. I told her she must be cleaning her own bottom because there was no evidence of anyone cleaning his small condo. She got upset with me and called me names, but I couldn't have cared less. I was furious that my father was living in squalor, and she was sanctioning it.

I was very sad when my father passed away because a piece of me died with him. I thought of everything my father taught me or gave to me. He was a troubled soul but full of knowledge. Unfortunately, in my opinion, he was unable or unwilling to establish meaningful relationships in his life.

Sadly, my father died alone. Nonetheless, I could not bring myself to cry at his funeral. In fact, during the eulogy at the memorial service, I joked about how he was an absentee parent. Some attending his service did not appreciate my humor or lightheartedness, but I did not care. My sisters and mother were there and, truthfully, I did it to entertain them.

One of my father's old girlfriends came up to me after the service and asked if I remembered her. I recalled that my father really liked her. At the time, she was still a good friend of the family. I had seen her when I visited earlier in the year.

I recall how she hovered over me for the longest time. I guess she expected a hug or kiss or something more than the handshake I extended. I sat there looking at her quizzically for the longest time before finally asking, "What do you want me to do, a backflip or something?" My sister Marie laughed out loud and then went and told my mother what I had said to this woman. My mother laughed, but you could tell she did not approve.

The funeral was much like others I had attended before. The only difference was that a calmness came over me that I had never experienced before. Not once did I feel like crying that day. In fact, I did not cry about or mourn my father's death until months later.

I still miss the old guy, even though he was a bit of a loner and went about life on his own terms. When I think of him, I can recall only a few memories of us together. I remember the time we threw a football in the park. That was our most memorable Hallmark moment.

I also remember the time he beat the crap out of my mother. I was scared half to death because I thought he was going to kill her. Their argument stemmed from his jealousy. Apparently, he thought my mother was making eyes at another man at a party they had attended. His pride was hurt. He beat her unmercifully for more than an hour.

I remember lying in my bed with the covers over my head, sobbing uncontrollably as if he were beating me. I never respected my dad from that day forward. I loved him the way a son loves his father, but I never respected him.

My mother triggered another memory of my father. It was a Saturday morning in Providence during the fall of 1972, and the leaves were a perfect burnt orange. The air was crisp, making it a perfect fall day. My mother woke all six children and piled us into her 1966 Chevy. It was not like we were heading to IHOP for breakfast; you could tell my mother was distraught. The only thing she said as we drove to Roger Williams Projects was "I want to show you all what your father is about." At that point we wondered where he was; we knew his car was not at home when we left.

We arrived at Roger Williams Projects, which looked like every other housing project in America. The buildings were constructed out of large, red brick. Each contained about twenty units, all in perfect alignment for about three or four city blocks. Even the projects looked beautiful that fall morning. My mother pulled up next to my father's 1971 Cadillac. It was a beautiful car. My father had exceptional mechanical skills and always maintained his own cars.

My father kept his automobile showroom clean. His car looked out of place parked there at the projects. The first thought was that it had been stolen and placed in the housing project parking lot.

My mother got out of her car and opened the trunk. She pulled out a tire iron and proceeded to smash all the windows in my father's car. We all sat inside her car and watched in disbelief as she destroyed every piece of glass on his car. It was early in the morning, so the sound was loud and echoed, yet no one seemed to be disturbed.

A security guard working on the property did see my mother, but his common sense told him to stay away. However, the guard trailed us as my mom drove back home. As soon as we got home, my mother called the police, anticipating how my father would react. The police said they could not respond unless there was a problem. Moments later, there was a problem.

My father returned home in his car with the broken windows. Because of my mother's phone call, a police officer had parked across the street from our house. The officer spotted my father as he drove up. He approached my dad and persuaded him to leave without creating an incident. My father peacefully came inside, and I helped him gather his clothes. He then left quietly as the officer stood guard outside.

Another memory of my dad was when his father died back in Camden, New Jersey. I had never met my grandfather; I had only seen pictures of him. Apparently, he had been very strict.

My mother agreed to attend his funeral, and my father said he would be there, too. I boarded a Greyhound bus with my mother and sisters Sheila and Debbie to make the trip to Camden. My mother did not have a lot of money but felt obligated to make the trip anyway.

We arrived in Camden, but the surprise was that my father never did. My mother was furious, especially since she had to borrow money from my uncle to get back home. I think she expected that we would get a ride back home with my father.

I was only ten years old, but even then I thought my father was a jerk for not attending his own father's funeral. He also wouldn't attend his daughter's funeral years later.

I was disappointed that he did not attend my sister Debbie's funeral; after all, she was his biological child. Believe me, there was no mistaking that—she looked exactly like him, as do I. People always thought Debbie and I were twins. Although we were only one year apart, she was the same height as me when we were kids. I did not have my growth spurt until the summer before entering high school.

It broke my heart that my father did not attend Debbie's funeral. You would have thought that he would feel compassion for her given that Debbie was murdered. We were all shocked by her death. I do not think my mother will ever recover from it. It was as if my mother's spirit had been taken, too. My mother began to attend a support group for parents of murdered children. My sister's death also prompted my mother to start attending church again.

My father did not attend my brother's funeral either after he passed from complications of AIDS, but I did not expect him to. My brother John was not my father's biological son, and the two never got along very well. I thought my father was especially hard on my brother when we were growing up. He would discipline him harshly, and treated my brother as if he were in the military.

I was happy when my mother told me she was going to therapy to help her cope the loss of my sister and brother. I probably should have gone to therapy for survivors of murdered family members. I never took the time to grieve properly after my sister's death. I had to return to the University of Memphis and finish my exams for my second year of law school. It was a difficult time for me, but I managed to pass all my tests that semester. My friends turned out to be a good support group during one of the most difficult times of my life.

When I learned about my sister's murder, I cried for hours. I had visited Rhode Island just a week earlier and failed to make contact with her. Once we noticed she was missing, the family feared the worst. It was not like Debbie to just disappear without a word. I felt like a private detective as I combed the neighborhood she lived in and asked her neighbors if they had seen her. She had a boyfriend, but no one seemed to be able to find him either. I left Rhode Island knowing I would return for a funeral; it just was inevitable.

I was dating a beautiful black woman at the time of my sister's murder. She also attended the University of Memphis. Jackie came to comfort me the night before I left for Rhode Island. We did not make love that night, but I had one of the most extraordinary experiences of my life.

Jackie and I were very close and shared the same type of goofy humor. That night, she was like Eddie Murphy, Richard Pryor, and Rodney Dangerfield all rolled into one. She had me laughing hysterically at her jokes and general goofiness. I have never laughed so hard or long in my life. We were so loud that my roommate Ronnie had to knock on the door to quiet us down.

I could have just as easily been crying that night, but I was not. It was another expression of the emotional wellspring that I was experiencing. I knew in the back of my mind that I had all this sorrow inside but felt an uneasy calm.

I was never good with difficult times. I avoided confrontation as a kid and never liked difficult situations. I still tend to shy away from confrontation. It has always been awkward for me during times of stress or pain.

I thought about my mother and other sisters and how I would comfort them. I felt helpless before I even got on the plane and was in zombie like state during the entire flight.

I was never big on small talk, and I was even quieter during those moments. I got off the plane in Rhode Island and one of my sisters and some other family members were there to greet me. My sister Sheila drove the car while I sat in the back seat with two of my nieces.

Beside Sheila was a tall, frail-looking person whom I initially thought was a woman. The person was wrapped in a blanket or shawl. It was not until Sheila said, "Aren't you going to say hello to your brother?" that I realized it was my brother John. We called John "Piggy" for most of his life. In fact, I do not remember anyone but the police or teachers calling him John.

Once we arrived home, I helped my brother up to his room, which had been my room while growing up. For some reason, my mother's house looked so small. I could not believe that we all lived in this small house with four little bedrooms and only one bathroom. Being there and seeing it again brought back memories.

I vividly remembered waking up in the morning when I was in high school and peeing outside because it seemed like either one of my four sisters or my mother was always in the bathroom.

Anyway, I helped my brother to his bed. He only weighed about eighty pounds. I just collapsed on top of him and began sobbing. I could not believe how skinny and weak he was. It was appalling just to look at him. He cried with me for what seemed like hours. I was overcome with grief because I knew this would be the last time I would see him alive. We read some passages from the Bible for a while, and he went to sleep.

I would read more Bible passages with him the entire time that I was home. We laughed, cried, and laughed some more. My brother apologized for all the pain he had caused me while I was growing up. He didn't know until then how much I loved and respected him. He was my big brother—stronger, wiser, and a fighter, figuratively and literally.

My brother never lost a fight in his life. He was the most determined person I had ever known. We would fight, and he would beat me up pretty badly every single time. He would crush me even though I grew taller than him and had a longer reach. He was always stronger than me. Even when we boxed with gloves on, I definitely felt the heavy hits to my head and body.

The only time I beat my brother in anything was when we played basketball. I was one of the best basketball players in my neighborhood.

I was about twelve years old when I first beat my brother at basketball. We were playing outside on the street with a makeshift hoop; someone had put up a backboard and goal on a telephone pole. That pole claimed its share of chipped teeth, bruised elbows, and face lacerations. It was dangerous playing on that hoop, which was about nine feet above the street.

There were two dangerous obstacles to navigate when you played at this hoop. First, there was the pole. If you drove for a lay-up, you likely would hit the pole in some way. Second, there was the curb below the telephone pole. You had an 80 percent chance of breaking your ankle on the curb if you were not careful. When you are kids, you rarely consider the dangers of what you are doing.

One day, my brother and I started a game of Twenty-One. It was early in the contest, and several of his friends gathered around. I was killing him. I had height and speed on my brother and began to exploit those advantages. His friends howled and laughed as I took him to the hoop over and over or rained jumper after jumper in his face. One of his friends yelled out "witness!" as I stretched out my lead. I beat him something like twenty-one to ten, which was domination for this game.

My brother was mad about losing. He took the ball and threw it at my face, smashing my nose. I began bleeding profusely, a faucet of blood gushing from my face.

I cried because of the blood; the blow really did not hurt more than it stunned me. His friends laughed at him even more. I ran home crying and holding my shirt against my nose. If I could have smiled, I would have because I had defeated my brother in basketball. I did not think I would ever beat him at anything, and I had beaten him at basketball—the game he had introduced me to.

Piggy and I fought often, resulting in chipped teeth, black eyes, cuts, bruises, and bloody noses. Piggy was a scrapper. He won every fight I ever saw him get into, and he always had the courage to fight. It did not matter that many times there was no valid cause. If a person disagreed with my big brother, it would be settled with blows.

I never liked to fight myself. That was evident by the two schoolyard brawls I lost when I was a kid. I had to survive the ridicule and shame of losing a fist fight with a white boy while attending middle school. Jimmy, who was about my size, kicked my butt in front of a predominately black student body. This was particularly painful because it happened during the airing of the television blockbuster *Roots*. Most blacks were on edge during that time. It's like you would watch and episode of Roots and instantly you channeled your inner Nat Turner. Roots was one of the biggest television events in history, breaking records for viewership at the time.

Jimmy was a good kid, and we were goaded into fighting each other by the biggest instigator in the history of Providence public schools. Another irony of that fight was that years later, I would date a girl who had watched that fight from her house. She even identified me as that kid who got beat up by a white boy.

Jimmy and I became friends after our tussle, but I am sure Jimmy always felt superior to me because he beat me up.

My other fight was with a neighborhood friend, Larry. It started like most fights do as kids: something of mine that he wouldn't give back. Larry kept my baseball, which he had borrowed. When he said I wouldn't get it back, we had no choice but to go to blows to settle it, right?

Our fight happened at a neighborhood recreation center, sanctioned by the counselors running it. We were both called down to a stairwell, and all the kids gathered around and watched as Larry put all kinds of lumps on my head. Larry was black too, and the counselors made us shake hands after we fought. He bloodied my lip and gave me a huge black eye, which I wore as a badge of honor at school the next day.

Thus, my fighting career was over by the age of twelve. I retired with a record of 0-2. I am not sure why I didn't get into fights after that because I had many opportunities. By that time, however, my poor pugilistic skills were known, and friends protected me from further shame and ridicule. Actually, I learned the art of dodging a whooping by using humor.

I had many friends in high school, college, and the military who came to my aid whenever there was trouble. I have seen some brutal fights both as a child and an adult. I never liked watching people fight, except for boxing, because I knew that it wouldn't resolve anything.

I loved my big brother for his tenacity. I sometimes feign having that trait because I admire it so much. My brother did not have it easy, though. Looking back, I realize many people misunderstood him, including me.

Piggy always had something to prove to the world. He was crafty but in a criminal way. He and a friend stripped copper piping from a home my family had been renting after we moved out. My mother was furious. Another time, Piggy and Debbie stole money out of a neighbor's car. The neighbor left a jar full of coins inside. There must have been more than fifty dollars inside because Piggy and Debbie were spending cash like they had hit the lottery. They bought ice cream and candy for everyone in the neighborhood.

Piggy's tenacity scared me at times. He was hell on wheels when he was angry. If I made him mad, he would chase me for hours just to beat me up. I would run from him and hide behind parked cars to avoid him. It was like watching a Saturday morning cartoon. We would literally be running around all the parked cars in the neighborhood. I would no sooner get to a parked car to catch my breath when he would catch up, and I would have to take off running to the next parked car. This would go on for blocks until I made it back to our house.

The most frightening moment of my life happened when I was a junior in high school. Piggy was upset because my mother would not give him money to buy the brand of sneakers he wanted. He went into our house and trashed the place. My mother came home and tried to get him to stop. Piggy threw steak knives and dishes at her, breaking even more stuff in the process.

That was a tough night in the Bean household. My mother cried for hours, and I remember having my first serious talk with her. I kneeled down beside my mother's bed and told her I loved her and that I was sorry for her. I said everything would be all right.

I began crying, too, and felt sad that she was going through such trauma with her own child. That night, I vowed to my mother that I would do really well and take her away from all this pain.

The heart-to-heart talk with my mother felt like a scene from a Movic of the Week. My family did not really show affection. I can remember my mother kissing or hugging me only a few times, and my father never hugged me.

I spoke to my mother that night for the first time like a man. The words poured out of my mouth as if they were rehearsed. I spoke quietly but firmly. It was the first time that I felt like I needed to protect my mother. It was one of the worst feelings I can ever remember having, one of total helplessness.

I had many good times in that house, but there were also many turbulent times—times that scared me. I vowed that my children would not endure such trauma.

I met my now ex-wife through her stepfather. We both worked for a security guard company in northern Virginia. We were discussing his art career when he invited me to his home for dinner. They had a beautiful home in Fairfax. The spacious house sat on a corner lot and had a nice, eclectic feel to it.

When I first looked at my ex-wife, I thought she was beautiful. She had the prettiest smile I had ever seen on a human being. As you have probably figured out by now, I like smiles. She was very talkative and witty. At the time, I thought she was a teenager because she was thin and had the exuberance of a young woman. She looked like a model, with high cheek bones and fair skin, and she was tall.

I stole glances at her throughout the night as I spoke to Rick and her mother. They were nice people—decent, kind, and a bit country. I was immediately drawn to them because they were a family—or so I thought.

I liked the idea of a black family living together and being so close. My ex-wife looked a lot like her mother, who was also tall and had a nice figure. Her mother was nearly fifty and looked great. She also had a great smile and a twinkle in her eyes whenever she smiled. We feasted on Kentucky Fried Chicken that night and talked for hours about art, life, and being black in America.

It was a good night, which ended with them waving goodbye from their front porch. It was a scene right out of a novel set in the rural South.

I felt good that night. I did not think much about my future wife because I thought she was only seventeen or eighteen. It was only later that I learned she was twenty-five.

Shortly thereafter, her stepfather came into the security office where we worked and we conversed. Somehow the subject turned to his stepdaughter. He said she had asked about me. I commented that she was pretty. He then suggested that I give her a call, so I did.

Our first conversation was sprinkled with flirting and suggestive remarks. She was funny and we seemed to connect on the same comedic level, which was rare for me given that I always thought my humor was a bit off center. We both always laughed at the same things. We would watch movies together and laugh in unison at what others did not find amusing. She was such a beautiful person.

The first movie we saw together was *Fargo*, which later was nominated for an Academy Award for best picture, and Frances McDormand won for best actress. The film was directed by Joel and Ethan Coen. I won points with her for knowing the directors. I have been a fan of the Coen brothers since their first film, *Blood Simple*. I told Christy about their history of quirky films and that I thought they were talented.

*Fargo* did not disappoint. It was a brilliant movie, and we discussed it for weeks after seeing it. My future wife was impressed that I had chosen such a movie instead of a testosterone shoot-em-up blood fest.

I slyly placed my hand on her knee during the movie. She did not respond and placed her hand gently over mine. She was a different girl, and I knew there was something special about her. We were inseparable for the next ten years.

Like most people, I thought my marriage would last forever, but it did not. When it was over, I had trouble reconciling my thoughts. I felt like a complete failure. It was not so much that I loved my ex-wife; I do not feel that I did. I married her because I thought she would make a good mother for my children. I was right; she is a great mother to our daughter.

The worst day of my life—even worse than when my brother and sister died—was when we had to tell my daughter that we were getting a divorce. I had just landed a gig in a show on the strip. We were living in an extended-stay hotel until construction was finished on our new home.

I did not want to tell my daughter we were getting divorced; doing so was my ex-wife's idea. Therefore, I thought she should handle it. She would not relent, so I agreed to present the divorce to our daughter as a mutual decision.

We sat her down on the sofa in the hotel. My ex-wife and I explained to that we had something important to tell her. My ex-wife ended up doing most of the talking; I spoke only a few words. My daughter fell back into the sofa, covered her face with her hands, and said, "I knew you guys were going to say something like this." And so it was done.

We had to stay in the hotel another two or three weeks until my ex-wife found a place for her and our daughter. I would occupy the home that was being built. To my ex-wife's credit, she got a place in the same neighborhood where my house was being built. In retrospect, I should have backed out of the deal because it created a substantial change in my life. I probably could have voided the contract. It was a small home and not in the best part of town.

Despite my concerns, I went through with the deal and was miserable almost the entire time I was in that home. Groveling, I begged my ex-wife to take me back. In an interesting and ironic twist, I told her that I would kill myself if she went through with the divorce. I did not believe it when I said it, though; I was just trying to manipulate her. But when I was alone with those razor blades and my drugs, alcohol, and suicide note, it was poetic justice—or injustice, depending on how you look at it.

I think about what a roller coaster my life has been, filled with so much pain. But I also realize I am not alone. Part of life, however, is enduring and moving on no matter what pain we face.

I still think about my friends' suicides. I cannot help but wonder about the pain, physical or emotional, they felt before making the decision to take their own life? Did they exhaust all their options? Did they feel alone? Did they feel their lives were worthless? Did they feel that no one loved them? I had those feelings. I felt I could not live another day. I understand what they must have been going through.

# CHAPTER 11

# REASONS FOR DOING IT

*Here is the test to find whether your mission on earth is finished. If you're alive, it isn't.*

—*Richard Bach*

According to an article in *Psychology Today*, one of my favorite magazines, there are six main psychological states that may lead a person to take his or her life: depressed, psychotic, impulsive, crying out for help, philosophical reasoning, and having made a mistake. At my lowest point, I was dealing with three of these states. I was depressed, impulsive, and crying out for help.

In this chapter, I will discuss each of these states, why it's important to seek professional help when such feelings take hold, and how I overcame my negative state.

According to the Center for Disease Control, depression tops the list of why people commit suicide. With depression comes the added sense of suffering and an honest belief that suicide is the only way to stop it.

Severe depression warps rational thinking. The suicidal mind accepts the idea that the "world would be better off without me." It is hard to find fault with a person who falls prey to such distorted thoughts.

The problem with anyone suffering from severe depression is that he or she often will suffer silently, so no one knows about the plan to commit suicide. Nonetheless, I recall being in a severe state of depression but somehow still functioned normally. I liken it to being a functional alcoholic: the person can put on a brave face for several hours a day, but at the end of the day, the person's drink of choice holds him or her hostage.

I recall doing everything the way I was supposed to, functioning at a pretty high level considering my state of depression. Moreover, I was doing my stand-up comedy in a production show and making hundreds of people laugh each night. Little did my coworkers and the show's producers know that I returned to my home each night alone and wondering whether I would even see the next day.

I understand how someone can be suicidal but trick everyone into thinking he or she is fine. Because I worked my day job and then did my comedy routine at 10 p.m. each night, I had a good excuse for looking haggard and sluggish. When I told friends and family about my schedule, no one could believe how I pulled it off night after night.

Surprisingly, even though it's not an easy topic to discuss, I think if you ask someone whether he or she has contemplated suicide, you will get an honest response. I have asked friends if they have ever thought about committing suicide, and the majority have said yes.

I have found that one of the easiest ways to broach a discussion about suicide is to reference a recent news story. Many people talked about Adam Lanza, the young man responsible for killing twenty-six people at Sandy Hook Elementary School in Newtown, Connecticut. Also, the spate of teen suicides or the suicides committed by US service members is also open to interesting debates.

No one walks around and says they are depressed when you ask how they are doing. Even in my most depressed state, I could muster a faint smile, and say I was doing fine. I often deflected the conversation to my daughter. My face lit up every time I talked about her.

It is easy to understand why a psychotic person may take his or her life. There have been several highly publicized tragedies that bear this out. I mentioned one earlier: the Columbine High School shootings. Both young men succumbed to their malevolent inner voices that commanded them to kill others en route to their own self-destruction.

According to an article written by Christopher Putnam called The Unburden Mind, psychosis can strike seemingly well-adjusted people who can mask their destructive intent. Psychosis can be treated just like depression can be treated, but the therapy may be more intense.

At the root of the shooters' actions was pure anger and hatred. Both boys had planned murder and ultimately suicide for months before executing their plan. What is hard to believe is that they sustained that hatred up until that dreadful April day in Colorado.

The other event that comes to mind is the shooting by Wade Michael Page at the Sikh temple in Oak Creek, Wisconsin. Page killed himself after being wounded by police. While many would characterize Page's actions as a hate crime that ended six lives, I see it more as a person who again listened to harmful inner voices. I realize Page apparently had affiliations with extreme white supremacy groups. However, I still maintain it was a psychotic act, driven by a severe imbalance in his life.

In the end, his act of violence garnered media attention because of its racist slant. It was really a case about a troubled man who took six lives and then his own.

Some people commit suicide when acting on impulse, which is often related to the abuse of drugs and alcohol. When I was a teenager, others around me liked getting high or drunk. I never understood the appeal of getting so high or drunk that you could not recall what happened the night before. I always wanted to store great memories in my memory bank and call them up instantly. This was one of the main reasons I abstained from using drugs and alcohol.

Alcohol and drugs impair judgment in many ways. In the case of the suicidal mind, it could be the impetus that sends a person over the edge. Think of all the terrible decisions a person can make while under the influence of drugs and alcohol. How many women become pregnant because they meet a guy at a bar then go home and sleep with him, all because they were drunk? Think of all the drunk-driving deaths in this country—approximately ten thousand each year, according to the National Highway Traffic Safety Administration (NHTSA). We often become impulsive and make poor choices when we are inebriated, which can have serious consequences.

The danger for the suicidal mind is that the person is already in a state of depression. Extensive research by The Royal College of Psychiatrists shows that alcohol increases the depressed mood of those already suffering from depression. Alcohol coupled with depression is a dangerous mix and you can understand how a suicidal person could act impulsively and commit suicide. The tragedy is that the decision was made quickly, impulsively. If that person had time to sober up, it is unlikely he or she would have made the same decision. The greater concern is when someone is drug or alcohol dependent. I believe anyone with drug or alcohol dependency should seek professional help.

Drug and alcohol dependency can be a cry for help, just like acting out or engaging in other attention-seeking activities. It is difficult to determine exactly which actions are a cry for help; that is why it is imperative for parents to pay attention to their children's behavior. When behavior goes to the extreme or simply is not the norm, it could be a silent cry for help.

I have had friends drop subtle hints when they were depressed, as people generally don't blatantly say they are feeling this way. For instance, just like I did, they may say they're too tired or overworked but not that they're depressed. To me, the cry for help will come in the form of a behavior that is out of character for that person. Maybe he or she starts drinking for no reason or becomes more sullen and withdrawn instead of being outgoing as usual.

The worst feeling I had when I was suicidal was that I was alone. What was even more alarming was that I felt alone even when I was surrounded by people; I couldn't fully engage with anyone. The most interesting feeling I had during this time was that not only did other people feel insignificant to me, but I also felt I was insignificant.

The cry for help is often faint. You need to be mindful of any clues and try to take immediate action. Try to fully engage with anyone you suspect may be crying out for help. You may be their last hope.

One day I had a discussion with my best friend, Steve. We were talking about reasons we might want to kill ourselves. I know what you are thinking: this was a far departure from talking about Peyton Manning's quick release or debating

Major League Baseball's designated hitter rule. We both laughed about having this conversation.

Steve said there were two circumstances where he would consider taking his life: if he had a terminal illness or if he were sentenced to substantial time in prison. I agreed with his logic, so it does open an interesting philosophical debate surrounding the choice to commit suicide. Certainly the terminal illness debate has garnered a lot of attention in recent years, with such high profile cases like Terri Schiavo. I don't think I would consider taking my life if I were sentenced to prison.

While a person may have the right to take his or her own life, it does not necessarily mean that decision is the right one. Another extreme example would be the prisoners of Nazi war camps during World War II. It would take an extremely strong person to endure the day-to-day atrocities of those camps without considering suicide as an option. Perhaps some people's faith helped them to endure the atrocities they experienced.

But removing those extreme examples, we are left with the philosophical choice to live or die. Does this decision rest in our hands? I say emphatically that it does, just like any choice we have in life. We choose where we live. We choose whom we marry. We choose the type of car we drive. Why shouldn't we have the choice to live or die? We can, but my hope is that you choose to live no matter what obstacles you are facing in your life.

You cannot be surprised by the notion that we choose to live rather than to die; that is the entire premise of this book. The choice is always ours. It would be intellectually dishonest of me if I failed to discuss that it is a choice to commit suicide. I refer to the story of Judas in the Bible. Judas betrayed Jesus. Rather than face his comeuppance, Judas took his own life.

What if you were facing life imprisonment like Steve proposed? Would that be reason enough to commit suicide?

The famed movie director Tony Scott took his life amid reports that he was diagnosed with a terminal illness.

Is a bleak medical prognosis a reason to commit suicide? I would have to answer that question affirmatively. I think if a person is diagnosed with a terminal illness, he or she has the right to die on his or her own terms. I have already discussed this issue with my daughter. If I am in a coma or brain dead or if I am in severe pain with no hope of recovery, I want her to pull the plug. No one should have to endure pain or suffer for a prolonged period of time.

I understand there are cases where a person has miraculously awakened after years of being comatose, but those cases are rare. What I am speaking of is a dire situation where a miracle is unlikely. If a person consults with a therapist or qualified medical professional, he or she should be allowed to die at his or her own hands. The person should have the right to leave this world with dignity.

This certainly is not a defeatist attitude. In my opinion, it is more realistic. Remember, we are not talking about an individual who is depressed, psychotic, on drugs, or crying out for help. This is a person who has already fought the good fight and exhausted all other means to live a functional or pain-free life. There is little or no hope, so he or she certainly should be allowed to grasp control of his or her destiny by alleviating further physical or mental suffering. I truly feel this is an instance that can be justified. I am sure there are those who would disagree with me, but I am trying to present a fair and balanced view about suicide.

Finally, I believe some suicides are accidental. Autoerotic asphyxiation is the practice of cutting off the blood supply to the brain through self-applied suffocation methods while masturbating. According to a recent article by Martin Down on MedicalNet.com, there have been hundreds of deaths in recent years attributed to this practice. It is widely speculated that the American actor David Carradine died in this manner, although his family denies it.

Another risky form of this practice, oxygen deprivation, has become popular with teenagers. Teenagers need to be informed of the risks involved with this type of activity; education is the only defense.

I personally consider overdoses to be accidental death, even though they are oftentimes characterized as suicides. The majority of the time there is a suicide note accompanying anyone committing suicide by overdose. Without a suicide note, this is probably the most difficult death to rule a suicide because an autopsy can never uncover intent. An exception would be if an extreme amount of the drug was taken all at once. The CDC says it relies on the official autopsy report to determine cause of death. Hence, police rely on expert medical examiners to differentiate if a death was an overdose or suicide.

Again, absent a suicide note, these types of deaths remain clouded in mystery. I would be remiss if I failed to mention suicide by cop. This phenomenon was introduced in the 1990s. At first I thought it laughable on the heels on the Rodney King beating. However, further investigation does lend credence to this idea. A recent case in Las Vegas involving Justin Hoey bears this out. According to a story in the Las Vegas Review Journal, Hoey was an ex-convict, who did not want to go back to prison. After being cornered by police officers following a vehicle theft, Hoey moved a loaded gun from his temple and aimed it at the officers. The officers opened fire on Hoey, killing him instantly.

A person with some knowledge of police tactics can create a situation where a police officer likely will use deadly force. I mention this because, again, we are left with a huge question mark regarding intent. If I am pulled over by a police officer on a darkened street and exit my car with my cell phone in tow, the officer could mistake it for a weapon and respond with deadly force. The reason I find the term "suicide by cop" laughable is because it gives an aggressive police officer an excuse to use deadly force against an unarmed citizen. John Violanti and James Drylie write about several cases in their 2008 book, *Copicide: Concepts, Cases, and Controversies of Suicide by Cop.*

The phenomenon has been called suicide by cop since Violanti and Drylie published their book, and the term suicide by cop has appeared in news headlines a decade before that. It has also been the subject of a number of books and many professional journal articles.

Incidents seem to be more common. A 1998 study of police shooting cases in Los Angeles County from 1987 to 1997 found that 11 percent of those cases can be classified as suicide by cop.

Absent the video tape that was produced following the Rodney King beating, the police have the final say on how any deadly incident is recorded and later reported by the media. Rebecca Stincelli, a former law enforcement instructor in California and the author of a book titled *Suicide by Cop*, has interviewed survivors of such attempts and says on her website that these people indicated they wanted to be killed by police "because they could not pull the trigger themselves and they knew, when forced with the circumstances, the police officer would respond with deadly force." This is a curious twist that a person contemplating suicide can rely on over aggressive, poorly trained police officers to do their bidding.

The cynic in me always found death by cop rather tenuous, at best. We have all heard of a death caused by police gunfire that is difficult to explain. I do concede that the police are at a disadvantage whenever they pull over a vehicle. The truth is, they have no idea what danger they face from the driver or passengers. I simply feel uneasy with the theory of death by cop without some evidence of a prior suicide attempt. In that 2009 study, which was co-authored by Peter Collins of Toronto's Centre for Addiction and Mental Health, 36 percent of officer-involved shootings were classified as suicide by cop.

The study sample included 707 cases from the U.S. and Canada between 1998-2006.

It also found that in 19 percent of the cases, the person "simulated weapon possession to accomplish their suicidal intent."

Some other findings from the study, which the authors say is "the largest known sample" of officer-involved shootings:

- 95 percent of the suicide-by-cop subjects were male;
- 62 percent of the subjects "had a confirmed or probable mental health history;"
- 48 percent of the confirmed mental health subjects suffered from depression or some form of mood disorder;
- 87 percent of the cases had "suicidal communications by the subject at any point prior to or during the incident;"
- 14 percent of the suicide-by-cop subjects left a suicide note;
- 61 percent of the subjects talked about suicide during the incident and 79 percent of those subjects referred specifically to suicide by cop.

The debate continues to rage on about whether suicide by cop is a true suicide or a homicide. Another form a suicide that is debatable is if an accident should be classified as a suicide. Accidentally taking your own life is more tragic than intentional suicide because the person never really intended to kill himself or herself. Most mistakes, however, do not cost us our lives.

In the case of accidental suicides, family and friends are left with as many questions as intentional ones, such as why the person engaged in such risky behavior to begin with or whether the behavior was a cry for help.

Accidental suicides are heartbreaking no matter the age but are particularly difficult when they involve a young person. Most of the time, a young person simply does not have the experience to know that some risky behaviors can have deadly consequences. I will try to differentiate what I feel is an accidental death from accidental suicide. Children have been killed playing the choking game. This is a game where you intentionally choke yourself to a point of unconsciousness, and attain a sense of euphoria. The trouble is there is a point where you are no longer in "control" and risk asphyxiation. Another example would be playing a game of Russian roulette. While there isn't any "intent" to die, the behavior is so risky that death is inevitable.

By contrast, accidental deaths might be the following: shooting yourself while cleaning your gun, driving recklessly and dying in an accident, taking more pills than you should have without realizing it, sniffing too much glue, dropping an electrical device in the tub while bathing, carelessly crossing a street. The key in characterizing a death as an accident or suicide is it's difficult to determine the person's intentions.

CHAPTER 12

# SEEKING TREATMENT

*He who has a why to live can bear almost any how.*

—*Friedrich Nietzsche*

It is not easy to admit that you need help to fight off depression and suicidal thoughts, but it is imperative to seek help the moment you begin having those feelings.

No one is immune from having feelings of pain, helplessness and despair. Feelings of suicide are not confined to a certain race, economic status or age. Even celebrity status, and outstanding athletic achievement cannot keep people from suicidal thoughts as evidenced by the recent deaths of three 29 year olds. Paul Oliver, a former NFL stand-out took his life, as did reality television star Gia Allemand, and Disney star Lee Thompson Young. It is unclear why these three took their lives with so much ahead of them, but they did. This should be a cautionary tale for all of us to be mindful that worldly success doesn't guarantee happiness and peace of mind. Our lives are invaluable and should be nurtured and held in high regard no matter what "status" we obtain in life. We must remain in tune with our core, our essence, our humanity in order to realize complete self-actualization.

Comedian Robin Williams' suicide was very difficult for me to process. Williams had struggled with drug addiction, and depression for most of his adult life. I liked Robin Williams' stand-up and movie career. His acting in Good Will Hunting was nothing short of remarkable. He won an Academy Award for his portrayal of a therapist ironically. That role was perfect for Williams, and in some strange way I think he identified with that character more than any other he's portrayed. The scene that was most memorable to me was when he and Matt Damon's character cry and hug it out in his office. You can feel the pain of both characters shoot off the screen.

When I was married, my wife insisted I seek therapy because she thought I was depressed. I believe I have struggled with mild depression throughout my life, particularly after I entered college. I never wanted to seek help because I thought therapy and religion, for example, were for weak-minded people. Also, there was a stigma in the black community surrounding therapy. Therefore, I did not want to accept or even consider that I needed professional help.

Finally, I relented. My wife and I sought therapy to save our marriage. In addition, I attended sessions on my own to quell my anger issues. It was the best decision I have ever made.

I thought going to therapy was like in the movies: you lay down on a couch, and the therapist asks you all kinds of probing questions going back to your childhood. It was not like that at all. I sat in a chair across from the therapist, and often I asked the questions. It was hard for me to open up to anyone, let alone a therapist. It took me a while to feel comfortable talking about my life, given all that I had been through.

One of the central, most effective parts of my therapy was relinquishing control. In most areas of my life, even at work, I was the influencer and initiator. Even in sports, I was usually the team captain or leader. I was always used to people looking to me for direction and leadership. Therapy was different. I was there seeking help, and it was humbling for me on many levels. First, I had to admit that I didn't have all the answers and that I was lacking real insight into my condition. I certainly didn't have the tools to handle this problem on my own. Secondly, I had to trust my therapist's judgment that our sessions would remain confidential.

This may be the main reason for not sharing my true thoughts with my friends and family. I didn't want to be judged, scrutinized or thought of as "crazy". Mental therapy is cathartic in that there is a complete release of the truth. My truth was that I wasn't the Teflon man, who could deflect anything. I was suffering, and I had to acknowledge I was suffering before I could get better. As I sat in my sessions, crying at some points, and laughing during others, I could literally feel the weight releasing from my chest and shoulders. I was willing to discuss anything, fear, frustration, prejudice, hatred, confusion, pain, uncertainty, rejection, doubt, pressure, and frailty.

I exposed it all to my therapist, unedited, a tremendous release. I used to believe in the stigma of seeing a therapist. That if you were, then there was something "wrong" with you and that you were not strong-willed enough to stand on your own and solve your own problems. I turned 180 degrees on that stance, and now I'm the biggest advocate of mental therapy you'll find. I understand the virtues of seeking and completing therapy. I know how desperately I wanted to get well. I remember being weighed down by my depression and wanting to work my way "by any means necessary" to a better mental state.

Over a period of several weeks, I began to open up about my fears, anxiety, and frustrations. Ironically, my therapist helped me tap into some unresolved childhood issues. One was that a cousin had molested me when I was eight years old. Up to this point, I had never discussed this with anyone except my older sister. She was empathetic and understood because she had a similar experience.

The therapist got me to talk openly about that experience and asked if I had confronted my cousin about it. I said no. My feeling was that my cousin knew what he did to me (and to others), so let him live in his own hell.

My therapist made me understand that what happened was not my fault. It was my cousin who had breached a trust and was squarely at fault. The psychological pain I carried with me was so heavy because he was a person I had trusted and often turned to for guidance. Later, I would understand how so many children get trapped in these situations and are taken advantage of by a sexual predator.

Years later, I talked to my daughter and explained to her how she always has the right to say no to someone. I explained that she needs to tell me or someone else she trusts if anyone touches her inappropriately or makes her feel uncomfortable.

Here are a few of the signs I noticed when I was depressed:

- Unable to sleep or slept too much.
- Could not concentrate and previously easy tasks were now difficult.

- Felt hopeless and helpless.
- Could not control my negative thoughts, no matter how much I tried.
- Lost my appetite.
- Was more irritable, short-tempered, and aggressive than usual.

I had at least three of these symptoms at the same time. I lost fifteen pounds after my divorce. (I called it the "divorce stress weight-reduction plan.") Everyone noticed my weight loss and assumed I was working out or eating healthier; it was neither. I lost my appetite and was not eating at all.

I was aloof during this period and had a strong sense of hopelessness. I also was angry all the time. My emotions were out of control. I looked for a reason to pounce on someone if I perceived he or she had wronged or disrespected me.

The worst moment was when my daughter, who was five years old at the time, did not want to go with me one day when I picked her up from her mother's house. While driving away, she sensed my despair and told me, "You are not fun, Daddy!" That was when I knew I was at a breaking point and needed to address my situation immediately.

I was so hurt by my daughter's words that I turned the car around and dropped her back off at her mother's house. Afterward, I went to my house, crawled into bed, and just cried. I could not stop crying because I knew I was in deep trouble. Nothing made sense to me anymore. My own daughter did not want to be around me.

I think it's normal to feel down from time to time, and you should not expect to be a ball of positive energy every single day. Moreover, real depression can be debilitate you, making even the simplest tasks difficult and overwhelming.

You can overcome depression if you learn to understand the signs, symptoms, and causes. If you think you may be depressed, I urge you to seek treatment immediately. The following are a few of the more common signs that you may be depressed:

- Feeling helpless and hopeless; having a bleak outlook that nothing will ever get better, and there is nothing you can do to improve your situation.

- Losing interest in daily activities, former hobbies, pastimes, social activities, or sex; no longer feeling joy and pleasure.

- Experiencing appetite or weight changes or losing or gaining more than 5% of your body weight in a month.

- Experiencing sleep changes such as insomnia or hypersomnia (oversleeping).

- Feeling agitated, restless, or even violent. Your tolerance level is low, your temper short, and everything and everyone gets on your nerves.

- Feeling fatigued, sluggish, and physically drained. Your whole body may feel heavy, and even small tasks are exhausting or take longer than usual to complete.

- Having strong feelings of self-loathing, worthlessness, or guilt. You harshly criticize yourself for perceived faults and mistakes.

- Engaging in escapist behavior such as substance abuse, compulsive gambling, reckless driving, or dangerous sports.

- Having trouble focusing, making decisions, or remembering things.

## | WHEN THE HUMOR IS GONE |

- Experiencing an increase in physical complaints, such as headaches, back and stomach pain, and aching muscles.

Here are a few indicators that you may have suicidal tendencies according to the Mayo Clinic in Los Angeles:

- Talking about killing or harming yourself.
- Expressing strong feelings of hopelessness or being trapped.
- Having an unusual preoccupation with death or dying.
- Acting recklessly (e.g., speeding through red lights).
- Calling or visiting people to say good-bye.
- Getting your affairs in order (e.g., giving away prized possessions, tying up loose ends).
- Making statement such as, "Everyone would be better off without me" or "I want out."
- Acting calm and happy after being extremely depressed.

To recognize these warning signs, you must be self-aware and honest with yourself. I became concerned after the incident with my daughter. I knew then that I needed to seek professional help.

I also realized that I was engaging in destructive sexual behavior. I was meeting women via the internet on adult sex sites. I was engaging in promiscuous sex with strange women and prostitutes and even having an occasional fling at work. I was out of control because I honestly thought my days were numbered, so it would not matter.

Suicidal thoughts or tendencies are revealed in many different ways and have many different faces. Anyone who feels down for an extended period of time should seek help from a mental health professional. There are many effective treatments for depression that can help alleviate the mental strain and stress you may be feeling.

Friends and family also can be a great resource. You should stay close with them and share your feelings if you think you are depressed or suicidal. However, keep in mind they are not trained professionals, and most likely are not used to dealing with mental health issues.

If you feel helpless, you owe it to yourself to seek professional help immediately. Depression impacts all areas of your life. Being able to understand that you are in a bad place mentally then taking the steps necessary to improve your life is what's important. Seeking help is a sign of strength.

## CHAPTER 13

# DISCOVERING YOU

*Who will tell whether one happy moment of love or the joy of breathing or walking on a bright morning and smelling the fresh air, is not worth all the suffering and effort which life implies.*

—*Erich Fromm*

Thank you for coming on this journey with me. It's not easy to discuss suicide, and it's a topic likely to send most people frantically searching for another more palatable subject to banter about. I know visiting this place is sometimes dark and filled with somber thoughts. I hope that my words encourage you to see tomorrow—a million tomorrows.

We don't lead easy lives, and anyone who tells you differently is lying to you. Our lives are fraught with challenges and uncertainty. Even when we are at our best, we can fall short of our goals or be denied heartfelt pursuits. I recall speaking to someone once about my comedy career and how at times it seemed stagnant. I wanted to give up. After thinking about it, I realized if I gave up, ultimately I am the one who would lose. I would never know what opportunities awaited me in the entertainment industry.

I see life in the same light. The only way we lose at life is if we give up. Committing suicide is the ultimate surrender, the ultimate retreat or failure. Furthermore, it is not just a failure for the person who commits suicide—though the majority of the responsibility does fall on that person—the failure also lies with friends and family, therapists, and doctors, none of whom were engaged enough with the suicidal person to come to his or her aid and end the psychological pain. Please understand that I am not placing blame on anyone here. I am merely encouraging all of us to be more engaged with those we love by making phone calls, visiting, and hanging out and not just posting pedestrian comments on social media sites.

There is a call for us to be more attentive to each other, to get in there and deal with the hurt and pain that befalls all of us. There is a reluctance to be around friends when they are going through a tough time. We do not know what to say; we are unsure of our role or simply do not think we have anything to offer during this time of crisis. But you can offer yourself: your time, your ear, and your empathy. Think of the times someone's been there for you during a crisis. My guess is you do not even remember specific words or conversations, but you do remember the person being there for you.

We have every reason to live starting with understanding our worth. Understanding your worth starts with accepting who you are, and embracing it fully. I believe that some people who work their entire life to obtain a goal or great success, in some way feel they don't deserve it. If you've earned it, then you deserve it! I'm revisiting worth here because I truly feel it's critical to gain proper perspective on how valuable your life is. Your birth marked one of the greatest days in history. Seek out those who reinforce your worth, and distance yourself from those who try to manipulate you into thinking you are worthless.

I happen to believe that life is filled with abundance. It is our duty to find that which makes us happy and brings us true joy. Time with my daughter is joyous, playing tennis, baking cookies, and performing stand -up comedy all bring me joy. I'm fortunate that I get to experience each of these activities on a weekly basis. There is a beautiful scene from the movie *American Beauty*, where one of the characters is filming a white, plastic bag being tossed around by the wind. He explains that there's so much beauty in the world that it's overwhelming at times. I feel the same way about joy, pure joy. So much of it surrounds us that we must set aside mundane thoughts and actions, and gravitate to anything that brings us joy.

The definition of "family" has changed greatly in the past few decades in America. Family is no longer regulated to father, mother, sister, brother. It has expanded to include blended families, combining children from two separate marriages. Family now consists of gay marriages, and many of those unions are opting to adopt children. Regardless of how your family is constructed, it's critical to nurture it. As I stated earlier my "family" is my daughter in essence, and I do all I can to connect with her in a meaningful way. We have our family rituals of watching *Family Guy,* playing tennis, cooking together, and going to the movies on Friday nights. One of the things I enjoy most is having certain funny references that only my daughter and I understand.

Family can build self-esteem, and also destroy it in children. It is our responsibility to build strong, cohesive families, which in turn make for a strong, cohesive nation. It is within our family structure that we are first introduced to our worth. We are cared for, and loved unconditionally. We are given a role in the family at an early age, and hopefully taught responsibility. We are held accountable for our actions, and when we disobey there are consequences. The importance of building and sustaining a great family cannot be understated. When it's done right, we create solid citizens.

I cannot think of anything more important than living a purposeful life. When we choose that thing, that pursuit that we are most passionate about, we can expect great things to follow. I was passionate about basketball, my first love and I gained my identity by playing. I enjoyed writing, even as a child, and managed to work in journalism for many years. It also led to writing this book. I've always liked the word purpose because it meant direction to me, a path or vision of something to come. I even think of the word purpose when I'm playing tennis. Am I moving with purpose? Am I swinging my racquet with purpose? Do I have a purposeful strategy?

Purpose belies confidence to me. It means I'm on a path, and not to be deterred. This in turn becomes a source of discovery in my opinion. The popular rapper Drake speaks of living his dream in many of his songs. I like his message because it is one of self-empowerment. Drake is humble enough to recognize that he is nothing special, rather he has worked doggedly at his craft to reach the top of the rap world. He encourages others to do the same, put in the work, and see where it will take you. For all the criticism that rap music receives, some of it warranted, we have to also applaud artists like Drake who promote hard work and diligence.

Our purpose becomes our lasting legacy. What will you leave behind? I'm leaving behind this book and my story of sorts. I'm making my legacy one of care, empathy and hope for those suffering from depression. I'm making it my life's work to help those in need, and to assist in suicide prevention. What will be your lasting legacy? What are you passionate about? Are you pursuing that passion relentlessly? This is more than taking up a cause, although there is nothing negative in doing that. It's more about you, what you stand for, and how you will be remembered.

It's painful to think about men and women who have taken their own lives. What is their legacy? How are they viewed in light of how they died? I'd like to think that men like Junior Seau are held in high regard, but it is doubtful given the negative stigma that surrounds suicide. I encourage you to think of your legacy daily. It's a great mental exercise that will challenge you in the choices you make each day. What will you attach your name to today? How will you ultimately be remembered? My hope is that I'm remembered for living an authentic life.

Suicide is a final, irreversible act. Instead of leaving a true legacy, you will leave unimaginable pain and suffering for those you leave behind. I think one of the most underrated human traits is our survival instinct. Somehow, even in the face of extremely adverse conditions, we can navigate how to live another day. When we fail to tap into this survival instinct and the intellect to problem solve, we risk moving to a defeatist attitude.

I have always marveled at the human ability to adapt and thrive in just about any environment. Resilience is one of our greatest traits. Regrettably, not all humans have the resilience gene; that DNA is not encoded into all of us.

Besides the feeling of despair and loneliness, another common aspect of the suicidal mind is a sense of hopelessness. No feeling is more devastating than hopelessness. Being hopeless is a gloomy existence where the future is not only uncertain, but any vision you try to conjure up appears bleak.

Part of the challenge to avoid feeling hopeless is to create a full and complete life, one where you always have something to look forward to. We often are called on to take up or champion the cause of others. One of the easiest ways to get out of a "blue funk" and step outside of ourselves is to commit to helping others who are less fortunate. I have noticed that when I help others or focus energy outside myself, I have less time to brood or contemplate my plight.

Our own narcissistic tendencies surely contribute in some way to suicidal acts. I say this because the focus is inward with a disregard for external matters. I am not suggesting we should not take personal inventory of our lives and self-evaluate. It is always good to understand or gain insight into ourselves while seeking to improve our lot in life. One thing is certain: we will face challenges every step of the way.

I wrote this book in the hopes that it will touch the hearts and minds of those who are having or have had thoughts of suicide. While I do not think it is normal to have suicidal thoughts, it became clear to me that many of my friends whom I have talked to have experienced periods of their life when they contemplated suicide. It was shocking to me because these people, by all accounts, seemed to have it together and were living seemingly full lives. There are more than one million suicide attempts each year in America—that's a lot of unacknowledged, undiagnosed, and untreated pain.

I think of the people I knew who committed suicide: Holly, Timothy, Cisco, and Danny. Each death affected me in a different way, especially Holly's. I felt if I could have shared more of my life with them, then perhaps things would have played out differently. I thought if I shared more of my struggles then it would have humanized me, and allowed them to share more of their struggles with me.

I believe I tend to be too open for this reason. I readily share my life with anyone who will listen. I try to present my authentic self to everyone I meet. Some people are caught off guard by this and are visibly uncomfortable. I understand, but I continue to present myself, warts and all, as one friend reminds me.

I cannot run away from the topic of suicide. I believe it's the worst way to die. The act speaks to the desperation, despair, and suffering a person must feel to consider it an option.

I have a friend whose son recently committed suicide. I told her that I was not at all uncomfortable talking about her son's death. She then spoke in detail about how her son was despondent and aloof, but she really did not see any signs that pointed to suicide. He did not have a great relationship with his father, and she felt that may have played a role in his decision to take his own life.

We shared a few lunches and discussed her son whenever it was possible for her to do so without breaking down. I could see the pain and loss in her face. She was visibly shaken every time she talked about him. I became alarmed when she would say she wanted to join him that she really had nothing to live for. It was always hard to find the right words to comfort her, and I am not sure I ever did. I only hope it was comforting for her to have someone to talk to about her son and the loss she has endured.

My friend's plight reminded me so much of my mother and what she went through with my brother and sister's deaths. My mother was so shaken by my sister's murder, and I know she will never fully recover emotionally. Her spirit has been broken since that day.

I see the same vacant look in my friend's eyes and hear the despair in her voice when she speaks. It is hard to see, and it pierces my heart to listen to her speak, particularly when she says she is tired and wants to be with her son again. Dealing with loss is never easy, especially if it is a family member or loved one.

I have considered loss when it comes both to love and death. Both are difficult to deal with. I hit rock bottom emotionally after my divorce. Fortunately, as I began to survey the situation, I realized that I was not alone; thousands of other people have had to endure the same.

A close friend once gave me great advice. She told me to just focus my attention on my daughter that it was all about building a relationship with her. She was right, and I took her advice. The lasting lesson from this is that it does not matter what we are doing as long as my daughter and I are together. Although my daughter is going through her teenage years, we are as close now as we were when she was four-years-old.

It is up to us how we will enrich our lives, what we will deem important, or what we will value. Part of that enrichment is setting a compass for happiness and staying the course. We must establish a purpose, much like I did during law school. I realize I have an unconventional way of looking at the world, but it works for me. I think I am honest with myself about what makes me happy.

But, as I stated previously, happiness is not the end-all for me. I first consider my responsibilities and obligations, and my individual happiness is secondary to fulfilling those responsibilities. In fact, by fulfilling those responsibilities, I feel happier. I am content knowing that I positively affect those who allow me into their world and afford me the opportunity to be fully present for them. My daughter comes first and foremost. She gets me like no one else. She understands my quirkiness and vulnerabilities and fully accepts me for who I am.

I see my worth daily. I do not need to keep a scorecard, trophies, or platitudes. I finally figured out that my worth resides in my ability to be fully present for those who I am fortunate enough to come in contact with. I now understand that I need to use the power that is within me to positively affect those in my life.

What is most gratifying is the understanding that my gestures do not need to be grand, just human and genuine. I must accept my worth to comprehend how important my life is, both to me and others. The other components necessary for a fulfilled life are building a legacy and accepting that my life is not my own, but rather it belongs to anyone who depends on me.

My legacy has yet to be written, though it may eventually be this book and my dedication to suicide prevention. I will accept that legacy because suicide prevention has been at the forefront of my mind for quite some time. When I read about someone committing suicide, I feel deep pain, especially when it comes to teenagers and young adults. Their lives are often snuffed out too early; they never have a chance to establish a legacy. I firmly believe each of us must choose something about which we are passionate and pursue it relentlessly. In that pursuit, a legacy will be born.

People depend on you—get used to it. Dependence can begin at an early age. There are countless examples of teenagers forced to care for younger siblings when their parents abandon the family or are killed tragically. The longer you are on earth, the more people depend on you. This dependence should be viewed as a badge of honor.

Moreover, taking responsibility for another person's well-being is noble. The first time I looked into my daughter's eyes, I thought to myself, "I am now responsible for another human being." I had to be better, wiser, and smarter. I thought about how my decisions could adversely affect my daughter.

I always try to look outside myself and put aside my own desires before I make major decisions. It is not easy being responsible for another human being—any parent will tell you that. There is a certain amount of stress that comes with caring for a child, even though you love that child dearly and unconditionally. You also feel vulnerable because you know your child's life is in your hands until he or she becomes an adult.

I have never shirked my duties as a father; I have fully embraced that responsibility. But at my lowest point, I was ready to abdicate my role. In that moment of desperation, it did not matter what my responsibilities were. On the other hand, it was the responsibility to my daughter that ultimately saved my life. Realizing my responsibility as a father gave me a reason to live.

My message is clear: your life matters. It matters that we have an obligation to our loved ones to fight and live another day. It matters that we have been given life and all the possibilities that it holds. You matter in ways you can never imagine. You most likely touch people and they count on you, even if they never clearly communicate that to you. If you were not here, your absence would be felt by everyone you leave behind.

I want to be clear that I still suffer from depression. I almost equate it to being an alcoholic or drug addict. I know I have to approach life one day at a time. I have to remind myself that what is happening right now, is happening right now and is not a permanent condition or circumstance. Like most people, I have had my share of disappointments and setbacks. I've lost high paying jobs, had failed relationships, and made more mistakes than I care to admit. Navigating through each event, setback, has given me time to reflect. I've tried to find my inner strength, and power through each time. Sometimes I feel these events test my manhood and resolve. Fortunately, I've risen each time finding a source of strength and resolve that I didn't think existed. Thankfully, I chose to live and fight another day.

Choose this day, and all the days that follow, to be here, to be present, and to make a difference. Your life is not your own when you consider it is shared by all the people you come in contact with over your lifetime. While you may feel your life is insignificant and without meaning, that could not be further from the truth. Life is a gift, each day an opportunity to love, laugh and evolve. You have so much ahead of you no matter where you are in your journey.

Every life is important. Every life has a purpose. It is up to you to find out what that purpose is. Ending your life is not the solution; the solution is living. Have the courage to live, to contribute in a meaningful way. Trust me, I know because I have been in the deepest, darkest pit of despair. There is an answer to every problem, and there will always be a reason to live. Now go out there and find it.

Readers may contact the author, James Bean, at
jbeancomedian44@gmail.com.

Printed in Great Britain
by Amazon